Unfinished Lovestory

BASED ON A TRUE STORY

Deb Seevers

Order this book online at www.trafford.com
or email orders@trafford.com

Most Trafford titles are also available at major online book retailers.

This story is based on true events, but names have been changed.

Printed in the United States of America.

ISBN: 978-1-4669-8080-8 (sc)
ISBN: 978-1-4669-8082-2 (hc)
ISBN: 978-1-4669-8081-5 (e)

Library of Congress Control Number: 2013902938

Trafford rev. 02/15/2013

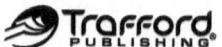 www.trafford.com

North America & international
toll-free: 1 888 232 4444 (USA & Canada)
phone: 250 383 6864 ♦ fax: 812 355 4082

Acknowledgments

To my wonderful husband and best friend, Ryan, thank you
for being my cheerleader and always inspiring me
to reach for my dreams. I love you with all my heart.
To my beautiful children, Amber and
Jasmine, I pray God will continue
to bless you in whatever he has planned for you.
I can *never* imagine life without you!
I love you both so much.
My family and friends,
Mom and Dad, I am the perfect model of you both.
Dad, you gave me desire to do my best,
determination to never give up, and bullheaded
stubbornness of a Gilchrist!
Mom, thank you for your tender heart, passion to give all
yourself to what you believe in, and the ability to forgive others.
I love you both more than words could ever say!
My dearest friends, God puts people in our lives
that we come to cherish, love, and adore, and I'm
so glad I have every one of you in my life.
Mel, Tina, LaGayle, Deb, Marty, and
the list goes on and on and on.

I can do all things through Christ who gives me strength.
—Philippians 4:13

Tears run down my face as I realize I can't move, and the soft glow of the recovery room lights beam into my eyes. All I want is him by my side, telling me everything will be OK. I don't want to be here by myself. Where is he? Before I can see him, I feel the soft touch of his hand as he gently strokes the tears away from my face.

"I love you," he says, and I know he does. But the thought of why I'm lying here brings it all back to me again. I failed him. I know I did. Hot tears once again race down my face as they create a pool of sorrow on the recovery room pillow. Where was God in all this? I begin to wonder if there is a god and why he is doing this to me.

We all come to a time in our lives when we wonder why. We doubt ourselves, we doubt our faith, and we doubt the reason we were created. Do I believe in miracles anymore? And do miracles really exist?

Once again, I hear him whisper "I love you." Does he really, or does he just know that's what I need to hear? All I can think to say is "I'm sorry."

Chapter 1

As I look in the mirror, I can't believe this is the day I have always dreamed about as a little girl. The dress is perfect due to the extreme talent of a mother who can sew like no other. The weather is perfect as all my friends wait patiently as I prepare for the greatest day of my life. Here I am, only twenty-two years old, and I know the man I will be giving my life to is just beyond the door, waiting to give his life to me. We met just a few short months ago, but I know he is the one God has for me.

We met in college, and after a relationship with a longtime high school sweetheart, I was wondering if that right guy was out there, or had I missed the boat of true love? Was it sailing away, and had I forgotten to buy a ticket to get on board? I know it's a really bad metaphor, but that was how I felt.

I was a typical college student—drunk, ha-ha—sitting at a party, wondering why in the world I was there in the first place, when he walked by. His smile captivated me, and I wish I had gone to the party with him. Why wasn't he the one I was sitting next to, giving googly eyes to and wishing he was holding my heart in his hand? But oh no. His name was Ryan, and I had seen him in class and thought, with a very evil smile, remembering him as he walked by and thinking, *Nice butt.* I know, childish, but hey, I was horny, young, stupid, and looking for any guy to take my mind off the roller-coaster relationship I had had for three years. As I sat there, pretending this party was *so* much fun, I looked over and saw him look at me and not with those eyes of "Hello, I want to be your friend," but "HELLO, I really want to be your friend."

He was cute and had a sideways grin that made me melt inside. I kept looking at him, hoping he wouldn't see me staring at him. He had gone alone, thank goodness. So why was he there? I noticed he wasn't drinking. I kept taking a drink, thinking it would help build up the courage I had, to ask him for a ride home, knowing that if I did drive home, you would be reading about me in the papers the next day. "College student runs over street sign and destroys private property." I had had offers from other guys there, especially Lance—nice, but annoying.

As I rejected help after help from others, I saw he was watching me. My skin became clammy, and my heart raced, knowing he was watching me. Why was he watching me? I was just a little country girl. I didn't think I was much to look at, but hey, when you see yourself in the mirror every day, the image gets a little fuzzy after a few drinks.

I could feel myself getting weaker and weaker, knowing that either I was going to be spending the night on this couch or I would have to find a ride home. And as if on cue, here he came. I could see in his eyes he had an intention of sitting next to me. Wow, he was sitting next to me, this country girl who only wanted to be loved by someone special.

"Hi," he said, and my heart melted. He was so beautiful, and to say that about a guy seems silly, but he was. His hair flowed sweetly over his ears, long in the back. "Do you need a ride home?" he asked. How could this be happening? Were the dating gods on my side tonight, or was I just getting lucky? My eyes swam as I knew the last few beers were taking their toll on my body as I said a hushed "Yes, please."

Knowing he couldn't walk me back up the stairs of Fryer Hall, I sat in his truck, wondering what he was going to do with me. Was he a noble man who respected women? Or the kind who loved them and left them? He contemplated for a very short time and zoomed away from the parking lot, with me inside. In his newly remodeled '66 Ford truck, he was country too.

Chapter 2

The next thing I knew, he was gracefully carrying me into a house I didn't recognize, seeing a strange dog I didn't know. But hey, he had to be OK. He had a dog, right? Why was he bringing me here, and whose house was this? I wasn't so far gone that I didn't know this couldn't be his house. He was in college, and this didn't look like a college guy's house. It was sweet and comfortable. Most college guys' homes were either filled with empty beer cans, underwear strung from the fact most guys don't know what a laundry hamper is, and the smell of rotten pizza they were too lazy to throw away. But he wasn't like those guys. His eyes smiled at me. Has he tried to get information from me? "Do you want me to take you back to the dorm?" he asked with a sweet voice. *No* was all I could think of. I didn't want to leave him. He gently sat me on the couch. Instinctively, my head fell on the armrest as I looked at him in amazement. Why did he pick me up, and why did he bring me here? I was aware enough that my clothes were still intact, and I could tell, that was never his intention. "You can stay here, if you want to," he said as I tried to get myself out of the chair.

"Yes, you better take me back," I said as I fell back into his arms, knowing far too well it would take both of them to get me out of the house.

I felt quite foolish, really. This is not the way I wanted him to see me. So I slumped back on the couch and said, without thinking, "I want to stay here with you." He smiled that wide-eyed grin that made me feel like a love-struck fourteen-year-old who had never been kissed. He brushed the hair from my face as he told me it would be OK to stay.

I sat up quickly, startling both of us, when it came to me—my car. My parents had just bought me that car, and if anything would happen to it, I would hate to see the look on my dad's face. "Don't worry, I have taken care of it," he said with a fatherlike voice. Apparently, he had a friend drive it back to the dorms while he was attending to my drama. How could he like a person like me? Drunk, stupid, irresponsible. He continued looking at me as if to say, "I'm here to take care of you now." Really, how could I be so lucky, and was this night one of those really good dreams you wake up from, thinking, "Damn, I wish I was still dreamin'"? But it wasn't; it was real. As I reached up to touch his face, he kissed me on the forehead, and my eyes fell shut.

Chapter 3

Oh, my head hurt. My eyes slowly came to life. I looked around, wondering where the hell I was. Oh yeah . . . Ryan's house. But where was he? I felt so foolish and dumb. How could he possibly like someone like me? I peeled myself off the couch. What time was it? I looked at a clock that I heard ticking in the distance, and it said five thirty. Oh my goodness! I slept in a house I didn't know and let a guy bring me to his home, but at least all my clothes were on. "You are so stupid," I kept telling myself. Before anyone could see me, I quietly snuck out the back door, past a dog I vaguely remember from last night, and began the small walk back to the dorm.

I really liked him, but after last night, there is no way he could possibly want a girl like me. I hope I don't see him in the hall that day, knowing that I would see in his eyes what a disappointment I was. I was very grateful the dorms weren't very far away, and the walk was actually good for me to clear my head and help me focus on the fact that I was a screwup. Ryan was going to be a memory, and that was all there was to it. A very sweet memory, but nonetheless, a memory.

As I crept into my dorm room, Mindy, my suite mate, began to yell at me. "Where the hell have you been?" Oh, my head hurt so bad, and I didn't need her yelling at me. I already felt like a tramp and a drunker loser.

"I slept at a friend's house." I know she wouldn't believe me because she knew all my friends.

"I was ready to call the cops this morning," she quickly began. Seeing the look of worry on her face, I realized what she must have felt, knowing I wasn't in my bed this morning. As she quietly—thank goodness!—questioned me about my new friend, I quickly thought, *Well . . . he's probably not a friend anymore.* Mindy wanted information about the night. She knew I had been to a party the night before because she was there too. But she left with Jonathan. Jonathan was sweet to her. He swore she walked on water. Why couldn't I have a relationship like that?

After the bombardment of questions, I finally told her whose house I slept at—Ryan's.

She couldn't help but get that smug look on her face, wanting detailed information about the night. All I could do was hang my head and tell her what I fool I had been. I was just thankful I hadn't thrown up on him or something really bad. I told her how he was like a knight in shining armor, rescuing me from a surely disastrous evening.

As the memories of the evening came back to me slowly, the phone rang.

Nobody ever called me unless it was my overprotective mother, and well, it was a Saturday morning, and I'm not sure why: because I hadn't gone home again this weekend. I just didn't want to tell her that I had been out all night with someone I barely knew and hear the standard lecture of safe sex, what would Jesus do? You know how it goes. So I answered the phone with quiet reluctance.

"Hello," I said, knowing the exasperating questions would soon begin.

"Hello . . . is this Debra?" the concerned voice on the other line sounded.

"Yes, it is . . . Who is this?" I said, trying to figure who in the hell would be calling me so early in the morning except for my mother.

"This is Ryan . . ."

OH MY god. This can't be happening, and how did he get my number and so quickly?

He said, sweetly concerned, "I was just worried about you. You left so quick this morning that I didn't get a chance to talk to you." Oh my goodness, how humiliating! I just knew he would be a memory—oh, a sweet memory—but there he was, talking on my phone, wondering if I was OK.

"Yes, I am fine . . . I am sorry I left . . . I was kind of embarrassed," I said with a wrinkled nose, thinking of the fact I had passed on his couch the night before. And before I could say anything, he began to chuckle. What the hell is he laughing about? God, I hope I didn't throw up somewhere and I didn't know. "Why are you laughing?" I said in a very timid yet frustrated voice. I'm pretty sure what I just said wasn't that funny. So I asked again. "What are you laughing at?" With a snide snicker in his voice, he began to tell me about his father and that he saw me sleeping on the couch last night. OH my goodness. How embarrassing.

"Yeah, Dad asked me this morning if I knew the strange woman sleeping on the couch," said Ryan with a giggle. I could only see the expression on his father's face, seeing the drunken mess passed out and slobbering on herself. Oh, I was soooo embarrassed. Now I know there will be no chance for anything. I could never face his father again.

"So that wasn't your house we went to last night?" I said, trying to get off the subject of total humiliation. I knew it couldn't have been a college boy's house—way too clean.

"No, I live in my parents' garage." What I was thinking was *In the garage? What is he? The banished child his parents refused to let in the house?*

"In the garage?" I said with same retribution of laughter in my response. "What, do you live in the car or something?" I asked him, thinking I was only making light of the situation and keeping his mind off the fact I was a drunken idiot.

"No . . . my dad built me a soundproof room in the back of the garage so neighbors couldn't hear me play drums." Well, that was better than the horrific vision I was thinking, about being locked away.

"Drums. That's cool!" I knew he had played drums because I had seen him in the college band. "So you sleep in the soundproof room in the garage, play drums, and . . ." I trailed off, wanting to say "With your mommy," but I didn't. I continued, "Maybe someday I could hear you play," hoping I didn't sound like an idiot.

"I would really like that," said Ryan. I could almost hear his smile over the phone. I knew he was really good at playing. I had actually heard many of the girls in band comment on his perfect rhythm. What they meant, I'm not sure, but I knew he was good.

"Well, I just wanted to make sure you were OK," he said with a concerned voice, but I could tell he was ready to end the conversation, which made my heart drain of life. I wanted to be there with him but knew this would be it; he was just being a good FRIEND.

Chapter 4

Monday rolled around faster than I really desired, and I was just hoping not to see him in the hallways of Vincent Hall, where I knew we had classes in the same building. I thought about going in a different door from where I usually go but thought I might as well get this over with: humiliation, embarrassment, and denial. About that time, my phone rang. "Hello," I answered, figuring it was Mindy, wanting to know where we were going to meet for lunch, but it was Gordon. Oh, Gordon, the three-year relationship that lasted until he went to college and decided I wasn't enough for him. He broke my heart. But to hear his voice was a comfortable feeling of the past. There weren't always bad days, but sometimes the bad ones outnumbered the good ones toward the end.

"Hi," I said, without trying to sound too excited to hear his voice.

"What are you doing this weekend?" he asked, trying to sound like nothing had changed between us, but I knew it had.

"I'm not sure, to be honest, and I know you won't be coming from Norman to see me," I said, trying to keep him from the idea of coming to Alva to see me and put me in another odd situation. Last time he had been here, he had been picked up for DUI because I wouldn't get back together with him, and apparently, he took his frustration out on a bottle of whisky, according to the officer. He wasn't actually driving when the cops found him but rather passed out in his car with it running. Oops.

"I really don't think it's a good idea. We are going in our own directions, and you know this is not what you want." I was trying to sound like I had it all under control. I loved Gordon, and in parts of my heart, he still had it, but I was trying to move on.

"Come on, Deb . . . I miss you." He was talking as if the sound of his voice would change my mind. And on many times, it had made the difference in my decisions. At one time in my life, I would have done anything for him. As a matter of fact, I did too much, but I tried to forget it. He was my first love, and I knew I'd never forget him, but times had changed, and so had I.

"Hi, Deb," I heard from behind me. I turned around, and there he was, standing, smiling that wide-eyed grin I had learned to cherish each time he smiled it, whether it was at me or not. "Oh, sorry!" he said, realizing I was on the phone.

Cupping the receiver, I said, "Just a minute," hoping I could have a few minutes with him. "Hey, I have to go . . ." I said, trying to get off the phone.

"Wait, I'm not finished talking to you," said Gordon.

"Please, I need to talk to someone," I said, trying desperately to get him to hang up.

"Who is he?" he said, with a harsh tone coming through the line.

"None of your business." And I hung up the phone.

By this time, Ryan had calmly sat on a bench close to the wall, trying not to be nosy and listen in on my phone call. "Hey . . . meet any strange women this weekend?" I said, trying to make light of the latest situation.

"Well, as a matter of fact, I met this very intriguing girl," Ryan said with a smile.

"Really? Is she someone I might know?" I said, laughing it off and trying not to blush at the same time. "I hope she knows what a great guy you are," I said, hoping he would understand it was my idea of an apology. He grabbed my arm and pulled me onto his lap. Oh my, did he smell good. I had heard he had a girlfriend, but I never saw them together, and I hoped he had broken up with her. So sitting on his lap I felt was OK. Boy, did he smell good.

"What are you doing later this evening?" he said, smiling that heart-melting grin. Was he asking me on a date? No, surely not. I was a drunken country girl who embarrassed herself by passing out on strangers' couches. He couldn't be asking me on a date.

"Nothing that I know of, but you do have my number," I said, remembering from earlier this morning. "Give me a call after band practice." I pray to God he hadn't lost my number. "You do still have it, right?" I said, trying not to sound like the adolescent fool.

"Yes," he said. Did he like me like I liked him? After sitting on his lap for a few minutes, I knew he was beginning to.

Then without warning, his hand began to caress my shoulder. I do believe my blood was beginning to boil at that point, and if I didn't get away from him soon, something bad might happen. As we were sitting there, Mindy came bounding around the corner and eyed my situation.

"Hey, girl, who's your friend?" Mindy was always concerned about whom I dated. She was my guardian angel in many cases. In my mind, I was trying to tell her to go away.

"This is Ryan," I said, hoping he would get the stamp of approval—not that I needed it, but it made life easier dealing with Mindy. It's not that she was overprotective; she was just a mother hen. I once told her that I swore I had moved out of my mother's house.

She always gave the look of "Deal with it." Mindy smiled at Ryan, and without warning, she did it. "So you're the one Deb spent the night with." Oh my god. She just didn't.

"Whoa," Ryan said, almost dropping me on the floor. Thanks a lot, Mindy. Now I'll never get that phone call today.

"I spent the night on his couch!" I said, trying to resolve the confusion and deflate Ryan's quick rebuttal.

"Oh, I was just kidding," Mindy said with her malicious grin. I could almost hear him breathe again. The reason I knew this was, I was holding my breath too. I so wanted to smack her.

"Hey, I will see you at lunch, and it was really nice to meet you, Ryan." She waltzed down the stairs. Mindy was my dearest friend, but sometimes, I really wondered about her.

"Anyway, about that phone call. I will be waiting," I said, trying to make him feel more comfortable.

"Yeah," he said as he went to sociology class.

I wasn't really confident about the whole "YEAH" and really didn't know if I would hear from him or not.

Chapter 5

"Why did you do that today when you met him?" I asked Mindy as we sat in the cafeteria, eating something for lunch.

"I was just kidding," she said, trying to make it sound like it was not a big deal. I could never be mad at her for long, but I hoped she would never do that again.

"Guess who called me today?" I told her, trying to sound as though it really wasn't important.

"Probably that idiot ex-boyfriend of yours." How in the hell did she do that?

"Yeah, it was."

"When will you ever realize he uses you, Deb? All he wants is a little piece of ass, and then he's off to do the next bimbo that comes along. Don't you remember catching him in his apartment last time you went to Norman and he had the gall to tell you it was nothing?

Wake up and smell the coffee. You deserve better." I knew she was right, but why did he have such a hold on me?

"So what do you think of Ryan?" I asked, trying to change the subject but really wanting to hear what she really thought.

"Well, he seemed nice, and I could tell he really liked you."

"Oh, how could you tell? You only saw us talking."

"Deb, I'm not blind, and for one thing, I could see the huge bulge in his pants where, apparently, you had left your impression from sitting on his lap." Oh my goodness, she could be so blunt sometimes.

"Really," I said, looking at her with a "Could you be any more annoying?" look on my face.

"What?" she said, playing off like it was no big deal. Maybe that was why he left in such a hurry after we had visited, or maybe Mindy just humiliated him. Well, deep down, I do remember feeling his excitement as we visited in the hall.

"He said he was going to call me this afternoon," I was telling Mindy, hoping she would share in my enthusiasm as much as I did.

"Who? The idiot or Mr. Wonderful?" she said, saying it in a way that was using her smart-ass voice.

"Who do you think?"

"I'm hoping for Mr. Wonderful, but in your situation, you never know."

"Yes, Ryan." I really wished she would stop with the sarcasm just once.

"What does he want?" Mindy asked, thinking I actually had an answer for her.

"I don't know." And I really didn't. I was hopeful, but after this weekend's events, he probably didn't want to introduce me to his parents anytime soon. *Hi, Mom and Dad, this is my drunken, countrified, passed-out girlfriend that you saw drooling on your couch last Saturday.* NO. I'm hoping maybe just a date to redeem myself. I really didn't drink that often; it was obvious by the lack of control I had that evening. I swear I only had three Cowboy Kool-Aids, but like an idiot, I ate the fruit at the bottom of the bowl. Someone neglected to tell me that was where all the alcohol was. Talk about naive.

It was three o'clock, and band practice was over, so I knew or hoped he would be calling me soon. Time passed like molasses, and by the time five o'clock rolled around, all hope was failing me, and I decided that his call would not be coming today.

As I stepped into the shower to call it an evening, the phone began to ring. I almost broke my neck, tripping on clothes all over my dorm room, trying to get to the phone. "Hello," I said, sounding as though I had just run a marathon on the phone.

"Hey, sorry it is so late. This is Ryan."

"Yes, how are you?" I said, hoping I didn't sound too desperate to hear his voice.

"Fine, I'm sorry for calling late. I know I told you three o'clock, but I had to work." Oh, thank goodness, a hardworking man.

"That's OK . . . I was just about to jump in the shower," I said, hoping he didn't think it was an invitation.

"Oh, I was hoping we could spend some time together tonight." Oh my, he wants to spend time with me. I'm hoping he caught amnesia since last Friday night.

"That would be great. Where do you want to meet?"

"Oh no, I will come and pick you up. How does that sound?"

"Great, what time?"

"How about forty-five minutes?"

"Sounds great. I'll be waiting in the lobby."

Fryer Hall had a great lobby with lots of TVs and games, but to be honest, I didn't want him to be in my room. It was a disaster, and I really didn't care. My mom always told me that if I ever married, he would have to be a very patient man and hire a housecleaner. Don't you just love the honesty of parents? As he hung up, I sprung out of the bed like I was on fire. Literally, my heart was. I didn't know him very well—actually, I hardly knew him at all, but the way he made me feel inside was beyond anything I had ever felt before . . . even Gordon.

Chapter 6

I think I took the world's fastest shower in the history of time. But I made sure my legs were shaved, my brows were plucked—there's nothing worse than a unibrow—and my teeth were brushed. Thank goodness Mindy wasn't there, or she would have been laughing because of the way I was acting. What was I, really, sixteen and going on my first date again? You would have thought so, watching me prepare for what I hoped would be a great evening. I even had time to paint my toenails and fingernails matching colors. That never happened.

He drove an old '66 Ford truck, and I knew he was outside the minute he pulled up. I really wasn't into vintage cars, but when he stepped out of the truck, I really didn't care about the truck anymore. He had on his Wrangler jeans with black cowboy boots—I knew he was country. But what was even better, he wore a Mo Beta shirt and cowboy hat. Oh my goodness. I was never really into cowboys, but I was quickly changing my mind. As I watched him walk up to the dorm, he couldn't see me, but I admired his swagger. God, he had a nice ass in those Wrangler jeans. As he approached the door, I noticed two girls admiring the same thing I was, but they made it a little more obvious, practically breaking their necks trying to get a better view. I just wanted to open the door and yell, "Back off, you wenches. He's mine!" But I held my tongue, which was a miracle in itself.

"Hi," I said as he stood at the desk, asking the attendant to call up for me. With such charisma, he turned around and melted every inch of my being with the trademark smile he possessed.

"Hi, gorgeous!" he said as he reached out his hand to take mine. I reached for him, as if it were an old habit, but knew the feeling shooting through my soul was something I had never felt before.

"So where we going?"

"Oh no, it's a surprise." Damn, I hated surprises but, in this case, was ready for just about anything.

"OK, but will you bring me back, or do I need to leave a forwarding address?" I said, answering him with my smart-ass comment. He just grinned his little grin and said it wouldn't be necessary today . . . maybe later. Oh my, was this really happening?

First dates are always the worst. You never know what to say, and it feels awkward when there is silence. But as the evening went on, I felt there was no time for silence. We were enjoying each other's company so much it felt too natural. He had taken me to a little restaurant in an even smaller town not too far away. As we were driving there, I made the comment that he was kidnapping me. He told me it wasn't a bad idea. I blushed, wondering if he saw the redness in my face.

Ryan was nothing but a gentleman; he held the car door, pulled out my chair, and even looked me in the eye when I spoke. Wow, I hadn't felt this special in a long time. Would this relationship end up like the last one? I don't think my heart could take it again. Gordon left a big void, and I was really having a hard time trusting again. My heart was fragile, and Ryan didn't know it.

"So I heard you dumped your girlfriend," I said, trying to find more information out of him. Not that I cared about his ex, but the farther away the ex was, the better.

"Yes . . . she was just not for me." That was a very political way of saying "I dumped her." And as rumor had it, he was now the best catch on campus, and he was with me. "Have you had any relationships?" he asked. I wanted to tell him what a jackass he had been to me and that my heart had been ripped up into a thousand tiny pieces, and I couldn't bear another relationship like that again, but I kept that to myself.

"Yes, I dated a boy named Gordon," I said, wanting to emphasize the word *boy*, "for three years, and we recently called it quits."

"Well, that's too bad," he said as I looked at him with confused eyes. "NOT," he said with a kidding grin. "So we are rebounding, huh? That's always interesting."

You always hear of how rebounding relationships never last. Never date immediately after you break up with a long-term commitment. OH my, I hope this wasn't the case here. I really liked Ryan, and it wasn't just his nicely shaped butt that made me want him. During our meal, he had made it a point to sit on the same side as me so we could be closer. Anyway, that is what he said.

"You are beautiful," he said as every inch of me turned a hushed pink. Was he saying things to get into my pants, or was he being sincere?

"Thank you. You're not too bad yourself." OK, I was saying that to get into his pants. I know role reversal. It's usually the male you have to watch out for, but he was so cool about not letting his feelings be known, until . . .

As we finished our meal, we walked back across the street where Isabel—the name of his truck—was, and as he opened the door, I could feel his warmth very close behind me. As I turned, we were face-to-face. He took off his cowboy hat and gently kissed me on the lips. You could have spooned me off the ground at that point because I was butter melting quickly.

"Thank you for going with me tonight," I said, talking in a voice of complete vulnerability.

"You are more than welcome." And he kissed me again. And just like the other kiss, I felt it in my toes. I wrapped my arms around him gently and squeezed my body closer, as if we were one person. His tongue was gentle and kind and played with my lips as we pulled apart from each other.

"Do you still want to go to the movie?" he asked. Deep down I wanted to tell him no because what I was feeling did not require us going into a movie theater. But I knew I had to show some sense of resolve. Remember, I was trying to redeem myself from the weekend before. So I said sure, knowing that going to the movies was the last thing on his mind too.

We sat torturing each other for an hour and a half, touching each other's arms. Gently caressing each other's fingers and finding myself wanting to throw him on the floor right there in the theater, not caring about those around us. But remember, redeeming myself. It was the hottest form of foreplay I had ever been a part of. He didn't really even have to touch me to send charges throughout my body, especially in places that were ready to welcome his presence.

As we drove home, we began making plans for our next outing, and it made me feel so good knowing he was thinking about the near future and not just tonight, no matter what it would bring. He apparently wasn't a "love 'em and leave 'em" kind of guy.

We pulled up to the hall, and like a scared little schoolgirl, I gave him a quick peck on the cheek and ran up the stairs. What in the hell was that? I looked back to see if his expression was as bewildered as mine, but it was too late; he was pulling away.

You idiot. I had the chance at getting another wonderful kiss from someone I was falling head over heels for, but oh no—chicken.

Chapter 7

Classes drug on forever, and I couldn't wait to get back to the dorms and see if he had left a message on my answering machine. I had left my cell at the dorm because I kept getting in trouble in class when the stupid thing would go off. So to save a drop in grade, I just left it in the dorm. Oh yes, the red light was flashing three missed calls and two messages.

I played the first message. "Hey, girl, I sure had a great time the other night and was hoping we could spend some more time together . . . Well, anyway, give me a call, if you want." If I want? Are you kidding me? That's why I raced to the dorm, looking like a track star jumping over curbs, to get this message I had been waiting for for two days.

Oh yes, there was another message. I hoped he was just missing me so much that he left another one, so I pushed play again, waiting eagerly. "Why are you ignoring me? You hung up on me the other day, and I just wanted to talk. I miss you. I love you, Debra. I'm coming to see you soon. Please call me back." Oh shit, it was Gordon. I wrenched my head back, thinking the mood had been shot. And what the hell was I going to do about this? I couldn't just ignore him forever, or could I? I told him it was over, but he didn't seem to get it. And when was he coming to see me? Could it get any worse? And should I tell Ryan about him? Would he support me on this or let me fight my own ex battles?

About that time, the phone rang again. I didn't want to answer it, knowing it might be Gordon, but then again, it might be Ryan. So I picked it up, hoping for the best. "Hello, this is Debra."

"Hey, girl. Where have you been?" he said, relieved.

"I just got your message and was just about to call you back."

"Great . . . I want you to come over to my house and meet my parents. They really want to meet you."

Oh shit. No. *Oh look, it's the drunken mistress who passes out in strange people's homes.* This is going to be great. "Really?" I said with reservation.

"Don't worry. They won't give you a hard time, I promise."

"Yeah, right," I said with a hint of "I really don't want to go" voice.

"You really need to come because my dad is cooking out, and he loves having company, and I would . . ."

"OK, I'll be there. What time?"

"Oh, six thirty would be great. And actually, I will come pick you up, if that's OK." What, did he not trust me, or did he think I wouldn't remember how to get there? You don't forget those moments in your life when you make a total ass out of yourself. I remember the street quite well—Church Street—because I remember I was gonna burn in hell for what I had done. "OK, I'll see you at 6:25, then."

Oh my, a date with his parents. Could this day get any worse? When was Gordon coming to see me, and should I tell Ryan?

I was waiting at the door at promptly 6:25, wearing a very simple dress, trying to not look like too much of a tramp, making sure all my parts were covered with plenty of material. First impressions apparently weren't good for me, so hopefully, my second impression would be tremendously better.

As we pulled up into the driveway, I saw a very kind couple swinging on the front porch. It looked like one of those Norman Rockwell pictures as they were holding hands and smiling like they didn't have a care in the world. Ryan opened my door and took me by the hand as we walked to the front door. I first met his mother, Janette. She was very kind, but you could tell she had reservations about me due to the fact she knew me as the midnight sleepwalker, and I couldn't blame her. And besides, Ryan was her baby boy; you know how moms can be about their boys. Next was his father, Mallory, as he gave this ornery grin about knowing what I looked like. I blushed again, thinking about the situation I had put myself and him in. Now I know where Ryan got his smile from. They were huggers; I wasn't. I thought this was the twilight zone. People don't just hug when they meet. I never gave hugs, or at least my family was not known for giving hugs and kisses. It was a strange feeling, being in that house, but they never mentioned my silly past the rest of the evening. Thank goodness.

After dinner, we excused ourselves from the table as he took me out to the garage. "Remember, I told you about my soundproof room. Did you want to see it?" *Sure,* I thought, *but wait, your parents are here, and isn't this really a little too soon.* I looked back at their expressions to try and find the right words to say. "Oh, come on. I just want to show you my drum set." Obviously, I had the wrong impression, and he knew what I was thinking. I hope his parents didn't read my face as well. That would have been another check on the naughty list for me. Two strikes—the third one, and you are out of here.

As we walked through their very large three-car garage, I noticed the black lab sitting on the carpet, minding his own business. "Oh, there is the mysterious dog I remember," I said, reaching down to pet him.

"Stop," Ryan said with a start. Immediately I retrieved my hand, thinking that, any minute, the dog was going to jump up and reach for my jugular. "Oh, I wouldn't pet him, if I were you," said Ryan with a lot of reservation in his voice. "He's been known to bite." *Oh my*, I thought. *Wasn't this the same dog I saw a few weeks ago and didn't seem to care I was anywhere around?*

"Are you sure?" I said, thinking he was teasing me.

"Yes . . . last time my ex-girlfriend was here, he bit her on the ass as she was walking in the door."

Oh, I wanted to laugh so hard but didn't want to startle the dog, Bo. "That's funny," I said, thinking, *Any girl who touches you will get a piece of me as well, even if they try.*

"By the way, how did you get out of the house that Sat. morning when you left so hastily?" he said, asking me and acting confused.

"Well, I walked out the side door of the garage while Bo sat on his carpet over there."

"No way," he said, acting as though that was an unbelievable thing that happened. "You don't realize this dog hates everyone but me, my sister, and my parents. Everyone else, he has bitten or growled at."

"Really?" I said, thinking the dog was smart and loved me already. That had to be a good sign, right? "Well, maybe that is a good sign," I said, laughing at Ryan.

"Maybe . . . he is a pretty good judge of character," he said, pulling me closer to him even with the dog watching; he still didn't seem to be affected.

"Either he doesn't think I'm worth getting up for or he thinks we are OK together," I said, hoping Ryan would agree.

"I think you are right," Ryan said with a smile. Oh, that smile.

Chapter 8

We walked into his room, which was filled with this monstrosity of a drum set. Quietly, in a small part of the room was his bed. It was obvious what he loved more. "Oh my goodness," I said, thinking, *Why in the hell do you need so many of them?*

"It's a hobby of mine. I've been playing since I was five." You could tell he had a real love for his instruments. "I used to sleep behind my dad when he played in bands." Sleep? How in the hell could you sleep behind those babies? I could also tell by the way he talked that he loved his father. It was so sweet, and you could tell he got most of his personality from his dad, but I could see a lot of his mom there too—reserved.

"Why do you have so many?" I asked, thinking it wasn't a dumb question, but I really didn't know much about drums, and then he began to play.

He had shut the door behind me earlier while I was admiring the setup and turned the radio up very loud. Immediately I saw the passion of drumming steaming with every blow to the drums. He was in his element. His passion was definitely drumming; you could see it in his smile. As he stopped, he smiled and said, "I've never let a girl in here before."

Really? I thought, beginning to get nervous again. Quickly the mood in the room became one of pure need and desire. "Come here," he said, motioning me to walk around the massive set sitting in his room. So I did as I was told and walked around. "Have you ever played?" he said, asking me as a teacher would ask a student.

"No . . ." I said.

"Would you like me to teach you?"

Right here, right now. No way. This would be embarrassing. I would make a fool out of myself again in this house, and that was not what I wanted to do. But in haste, I said, "Sure."

He motioned for me to sit on the stool, as he called it, in front of him. *Oh, this couldn't be good,* I thought to myself, and then, *On the other hand, it could be really good.* As I sat on the oddly shaped apparatus, he put his arms around me and put the sticks in my hand. But instead of letting me play by myself, he held my hands with his. The sticks were intertwined togetherness in our fingers. It was a feeling of complete control that I had over him. He was letting me play with his toy. So many erotic thoughts began to flow through my mind, and I knew this was going to be good, or at least I was hoping. As his hands touched me, I heard the music switch to a jazzier style of music, and we began to make music together. The experience was almost erotic as I felt him press on the bass drum pedal and at the same time felt the muscles in his legs push against mine. "I love jazz," he said, whispering in my ear. I was beginning to love it just as much. "I like it when you play with me." he said once again, softly breathing jazz into my ear. What was he saying? Was I taking this the wrong way, or did he mean what I think he meant?

His smell made me never want to get up again. I would spend eternity sitting next to him, if it provided the same feelings I had for the rest of my life. I could feel myself getting hotter, and I was hoping it wasn't showing on the outside due to the fact we were sitting so close together. I wanted so badly to turn around but was startled as the door swung open, and Bo, being the bad boy that he was, snuck into the room. *Stupid dog*, I thought, because at that point, all the air left the room, and the music had stopped.

As we were walking out the door, I noticed a wedding picture of Ryan and a beautiful redheaded woman. I thought to myself, *He's been married.* "So who's this in the picture with you?" I said, thinking surely she was family.

"Oh . . . she was my wife," he said in a meek voice, emphasizing the word *WAS.* I could have died right there. I felt so bad that I had even mentioned anything. I looked at him with sad eyes, trying to convey my sympathies, but then I saw the ornery look I had come to adore.

"Oh bull," I said. "Who is she really?" With a chuckle, he told me she was his sister, Cris. I knew I was going to have my hands full with this one.

And of course, as perfect timing would have it, a message buzzed in my pocket. "What was that?" Ryan said with a smile.

"Wouldn't you like to know," I said, smiling with my mischievous grin. I picked up the phone, and he could tell something was wrong by the look on my face.

"What's wrong?" he asked, knowing that I had bad news but not knowing if I would let him in on the conversation.

"Oh, nobody." Before I realized what I had said, he frowned at me. "I mean, nothing's wrong," I said, trying to hide the fact that he had not asked me WHO was on the line but rather WHAT was happening on the phone message.

"Do you have something you need to talk about?" he asked, sounding truly concerned, but I didn't want him to get involved in my stupid ex situation.

"No, I just have something I need to deal with, and I don't want to get you involved."

"Is it him?" he asked me with a hateful, jealous look. I still didn't want him involved with my past. I wanted a future with him and did not involve things that I had done in the past to cloud up the fact that I really liked him sooo much.

"Don't worry about it," I tried to say lightheartedly.

"I will worry about it. I don't like anyone giving you a hard time, and if I can do something about it, I will." It wasn't about not thinking he couldn't stand up against Gordon. Ryan had muscles in places he shouldn't have muscles. He was broad shouldered and had the look of a body builder—that was not my concern. As I was trying to talk to him about being rational, I heard it. "What's wrong?" he asked, knowing that I had a look that recalled fear, hatred, and anguish—all in the same face.

"Oh, nothing . . ." But I was hearing the sound of Gordon's Z28 outside. I had heard that sound for many years and knew it by heart. In his message I just received moments earlier, he had put that he was in town looking for me. *Why in the hell is he doing this to me?* I said to myself. *I want to move on, and who would want someone like me with baggage hanging around them at every corner?* As I heard the sound of the car again, my skin began to crawl, and I began to fear the worst.

"Is that son of a bitch at my house?"

I don't know if he said it because he was pissed that I had brought trouble to his family's home or if he was truly concerned about me. How did Gordon even know where Ryan lived? Who could have told him? Once again, I heard him go around the block, and I hurried to the side door to see if it was really him. As I stepped onto the lawn, he began to pull up onto the driveway. *Oh my god, NO. Get out of here,* I thought. *What gives you the right to meddle in my business?*

Quickly he got out of the car and began to move closer to me. "Go in the house!" *What?* Ryan had been standing behind me the

whole time and was watching what was about to unfold. "Please go in
the house," he said as he grabbed my arm slowly with true concern in
his eyes.

No, I don't want you fighting my battles for me. "Please don't, Ryan.
I can take care of this, please."

"Go in the house. It's time for me to take care of you." Did he just
say that? I hardly knew him, and he was ready to beat anyone who
wanted to hurt me. "Go!" he said hastily, pointing to the house with
such forcefulness, and I could do nothing but obey. As I walked into
the garage, I looked and saw that Ryan's parents' car was gone. Thank
goodness they would not be here to witness this atrocity. That would
definitely be my third strike, and I would be out of there.

"Hey, Deb, wait . . . I just want to talk to you," Gordon said,
trying to get me to come back outside.

"Who in the hell do you think you are?" I heard this as I leaned
against the door from the inside of the garage.

"Get out of my way, you asshole. I just want to talk to her."

"I don't give a shit. She obviously doesn't want to talk to you,
so get the hell off my property," Ryan said as he walked up to face
Gordon so he wouldn't get any closer to me or the house. Why was
Ryan doing this? He didn't have to fight my battles. We had only been
dating for a very short time, and . . . well, nobody had ever fought for
me before.

"Don't make me tell you again," he said as they stood toe to
toe, fury steaming from Ryan's face as I watched from the kitchen
window. But Ryan held his ground, and without even touching him,
in a voice I had never heard him use, I heard him once more say,
"Get off my property, or I am going to beat the living shit out of
you," gritting his teeth with every word he spoke. Gordon was never a
fighter, so he backed away, got into his car, and drove away, skidding
up the road.

Oh my goodness, that was the most intense situation I had ever
been a part of. I watched as Ryan observed him leave and go around,

down another street, then he turned and walked back toward the house. I stood in the doorway, shaking so badly, and all I wanted to do was hold him. Would he be mad that I had brought this to him, or would he comfort me in my state of horror?

Chapter 9

As I sat on the back step, I had tears running down my cheeks, and as I looked up, Ryan stood there with a look I had not seen in his eyes. They were burning with passion, but I wasn't sure if it was because he was mad and didn't want to deal with the issues that came along with me. Heavens, just last week I passed out on his parents' couch, exes keep texting me, and I am a basket case.

"Stand up!" he said, and I was thinking he wanted me out of his house too. I was so stupid to think I could ever have a relationship that would last. I am used goods and filled with drama. Who wants that?

I had my head hung low, and tears were really beginning to flow as they dripped on the concrete floor. He slowly lifted my chin with his warm touch and looked me in the eyes.

"I'm sorry!" I said as I started to walk toward the door.

"Where are you going?" he asked me with a voice that was so sweet and protective.

"You don't want me . . . My life is a mess, and you deserve someone who has less baggage to carry around," I said, trying to escape out the door with some dignity left in me.

"No," he said.

"No what?" I asked through tear-stained eyes.

"You aren't going anywhere but here with me." Does he really mean this? Why would this beautiful man need this drunken screwup to be a part of his life?

"Come here," he said with no reservation or thought and pulled me closer so we were touching. "I will never let him hurt you again. I promise." Ryan was standing up for me and was holding me—me, the person who felt unworthy of the most eligible bachelor at Northwestern. He was holding me.

He took me by the hand, and we headed back toward the room where we had just been just a few short moments ago, in his territory, in his safe place. He opened the door like a gentleman and motioned me to enter as he closed the door behind us. *What is happening?* I wondered, trying to wipe the mascara that I was sure was running down my face. I was sure I looked hideous, but once again, he looked me in the eye and brushed my matted hair away from my face.

"I promise you he will never hurt you again," Ryan whispered in my ear as he slowly took me in his arms. Gently he took both of his hands and cupped them around my face and kissed me with the feeling of security, and my body felt as though it wanted to fall through his arms. His kisses were that powerful. Each one felt like the first, and with every one, every cell in my body reacted to his touch.

"Come sit down," he said as we sat on the edge of his bed. "I want to show you just how much you mean to me, and if you don't want to, I will stop." *You want to show me?* What was that supposed to mean? Was he going to write me a love poem, sing to me? What?

It couldn't be what I thought it's going to be. I barely knew him, but I also felt like I had known him my entire life. And why would I agree to this? Because I had never felt like this toward anyone else, even Gordon. But this was NO time to be thinking about him. He was, hopefully, gone, and I was sitting with Ryan. His eyes held me mesmerized as he told me how long he had admired me from afar, knowing I had a boyfriend.

"I've prayed we would have this opportunity to share with each other. Am I surprised it is so soon? Yes, but I'm not about to argue about it," he said, thankful for what we were sharing with each other. "I want to make love to you, Debra, and not because we're here alone but because I have never met anyone like you, and I want you for myself."

I sat there thinking, *Please don't wake up. This is the best dream I have ever had.*

"But if this is not what you want, we can wait," he said, telling me this so I knew I could say no at any moment if I needed.

"I want you . . ." I said without reservation, and leaned into him to return the favor of his sweet kisses.

His hand slowly filtered through my hair as we kissed uncontrollably. Our tongues danced with each other in perfect harmony, sometimes fast and sometimes slow, but always in perfect motion. Was this going too fast? Was I making a mistake? Would I regret this tomorrow? At that moment, I didn't care and let what was about to happen take its course. I didn't want to let him go, I did want someone to protect me, and I was worthy of love.

Without taking his eyes off me, he began to unbutton my shirt one at a time, slowly enjoying each one as he went. As he pushed the shirt over my shoulders, exposing my alabaster-white skin, he kissed my shoulders and nibbled on my neck, raising my body heat from 98.7 to over boiling. *God, I hope his parents don't come home soon.* And why was I thinking about them at a moment like this? I know I didn't want strike three: premarital sex. Big no-no in my parents' book too.

His puppy-dog eyes were chocolaty brown and could burn through me like I were melted butter. He looked at me and asked if I was still OK. I responded with a sincere yes. I could see he liked control, and I didn't mind being submissive to his needs at that moment. Without warning, his hand slipped behind me, and within seconds, I realized he had undone my bra as I lay there exposed. He had obvious experience. Lying there, wondering who all those he had practiced on were, I thought to myself, *Well, the only one he will be practicing on will be me from now on.*

"Oh, Ryan . . ." I hissed as my back arched to meet his kisses. If this was passion, I had never truly felt it before in my life. Whatever I had experienced in my past was no more. I wanted Ryan for an eternity.

As he lay next to me, I could feel his erection, and I knew there was no turning back at this point. I took off his shirt as I pulled the hem of his T-shirt and raised it over his head, exposing his chest. I could get lost in his chest hair and loved the pecs behind them. He was so well built, and as I thought those words, he picked me up and sat me on his lap. "Wasn't this the first place you liked to sit?" he said, remembering the hallway discussion earlier that week.

"Absolutely," I said in a very quiet and still voice. My breasts were directly in front of him, and as he kissed each only gently, I threw my head back, absorbing every tingle it gave my body. I could feel him below, begging to be released from his fabric cage, and I obliged graciously, watching him spring forth like a caged animal. He gasped as I exposed him and gave me a reassuring look of confidence.

"Are you prepared?" I asked, hoping that what we were about to do didn't have to be abruptly stopped due to no protection.

"Yes," he said as he opened the drawer next to his bed. I looked in and only saw one, so I was glad of that. I wouldn't want to think this was his stash and I was just one of many. "Remember, you are the only one I have ever let in here," he said, reassuring me that this drawer was only meant for me.

"Did you know this was going to happen?" I asked, not wanting to spoil the mood, but I needed to know if this was what he had planned all along.

"NO!" he said, almost taking offense to my question. "I put it there in hopes of someday, but I never thought it would be today," he said as he kissed me again.

We made passionate love for what seemed forever and ended up on the floor, not knowing how we got there but not seeming to mind. After we were both spent, he reached up and took my face in his hands and sincerely told me, "You are so beautiful." *Thank you* was all that I could say as we lay there wrapped in each other's arms. I never wanted that night to end.

Chapter 10

As we put ourselves back together, ironically, his parents drove into the garage. *PHEW,* I thought as I buttoned the last button, and we walked out looking like nothing had ever happened. His parents had been to church—oh, that made me feel even better. Sinners. *Oh, but what a sin it was,* as I smiled on the inside. "You really should get a place of your own," I whispered in his ear, away from where they were sitting.

"I plan to. That's why I'm staying here," he exclaimed. "I've been here, saving for the day I want to put down money for a house of my own. What, you thought I planned on living with my parents for my entire life?" He almost burst into laughter but didn't want to explain to his parents his reaction. They liked having their baby boy close to home.

I thanked Janette and Mallory for a lovely evening and got into the truck so Ryan could take me back to the dorm. I checked him at the door, and we walked up the stairs to the third floor and into room

321. Thank goodness I had picked up in the room the day before, or he would really think I was a pig. I had put two twin-size beds together, and it pretty much covered the entire room. "We could have some fun in here," he said with a melancholy look. What a brat.

"Sorry, I don't have a drawer with special things in it here." He looked at me with a grateful look, hoping I was just kidding. "I'm just kidding, goodness. I will let you be a Boy Scout and always be prepared. How does that sound?"

"Good. I like wearing the pants in the relationship." He was smiling as he said it, knowing he meant something else. God, he was ornery.

Mindy bounced around the corner and said, "Oh, I thought I heard voices. Do you plan on spending the night here?" She was smiling that shit-eating grin she carried so well.

"No, but I'd like to . . . maybe some other day," he said, giving me a reassuring pat on the behind. Mindy's face was classic, and I knew I would be getting the fifty inquiring questions as soon as he left.

"Oh no . . ." I said, startling both Ryan and Mindy.

"What, for crying out loud? You scared the crap out of me," Mindy said, looking at me with the "what the hell" look.

"I forgot my phone at your house." How could I have been so stupid? It was already so late, and I didn't want to get out again. Plus it would be a great excuse for Ryan to see me again soon. "Could you bring it to me in the morning?" I asked, hoping he would get the hint, and he did with an amusing smile.

"It would be my pleasure," he said, almost making Mindy want to puke with his persuasive talk.

"Oh please. I know what you two have been up to," she said, holding back no sarcasm whatsoever. "Well, you don't have to worry about me. I will be busy myself, so don't bother me." Obviously, Jonathan was going to be in town, and she was sneaking him up the stairs for an evening of romper room. She's so crazy.

She always told me never to disturb her when Jonathan was in town; I just hope she didn't get caught from the school campus. They were real asses when it came to following the dorm rules. And lately, that had been putting patrols at all the dorms, making room checks.

So getting caught after hours would not be a good idea. Plus I knew Ryan would be returning the morning, or anyway, I hoped he would be.

Chapter 11

As I lay in bed, recapping the events that unfolded this evening, I couldn't help but smile. It was about two in the morning, and I kept replaying it in my mind, not helping me go to sleep at all but creating a desire to go back to his house, sneak in the garage, and do it all over again. I wasn't worried about Bo anymore. He was on my side.

I could also hear a faint sound coming from Mindy's room, and I wasn't about to go share any more information with her. We had enjoyed at least an hour sharing how I was head over heels in love but was afraid of saying it just yet. She was busy, and she hated to be disturbed except for emergencies only . . . ha-ha. There was no way I would want to walk in on that anyway. I knew she and Jonathan would last because he put up with her smart ass and she loved him unconditionally.

Thinking about tomorrow helped me control the fact that I would be seeing him very soon, so I began to drift off to sleep. *BAM BAM*.

What in the hell! Someone was at my door, and they were making it quite obvious they needed in. Oh, surely Ryan wouldn't be sneaking up here, taking the risk of getting me in trouble. It was probably Susie down the hallway. When she got drunk, she always went to the wrong room half the time, and one of us would have to direct her back to bed. She was funny, and she also walked in her sleep. Two combinations I certainly wouldn't want. Hahaha. *BAM BAM.* "OK, I'm coming," I said as I swung the door open.

"Oh dear god . . . What are you doing here?"

Gordon was standing in the hallway, drunk as a skunk. I could smell the liquor on his breath, and I looked down the hallway to see if anyone else was watching what was unfolding. "Get out of here!" I said with a hushed voice, knowing that if I got caught, I would be in deep shit not only with campus security but with Ryan.

"Please, I just want to talk to you," he begged with a rather loud and compelling voice. I grabbed his arm and drug him into the room, hoping no one would see him.

"What are you doing here? You know we are over, and you really need to move on." I pleaded with him to leave. I went to call security but realized my phone wasn't there, and I wasn't about to make a scene, not in the middle of the night. God, I wished Ryan were here. I needed my knight in shining armor.

"I love you . . . and I'm sorry for all the things I have done to you," he said, almost tripping over my chair.

"I know you do, and I loved you too, very much, but I don't love you anymore. Please leave," I said, wanting to scream it from the top of my lungs. Goodness, he reeked of liquor. "Where have you been drinking?" I said, knowing that there were three bars in town, and they were probably the sources of his loathsome drinking.

"What do you care? Please, can I spend the night here, then?" He was slurring every word he said, and I was having a difficult time understanding, anyway.

"No, you can't spend the night here."

"Oh, come on, it will be just like the good ole days." Yeah, he had to bring that up. I will admit it was good once, but that was then, and this is now.

"Don't touch me!" I said with just a little more venom in my voice. He sat on the edge of the bed, giving me a look of desire, thinking that I would just do as he commanded, but I held my ground, inching closer to the door that connected Mindy's room and mine. I didn't care if she was doing it with Jonathan; I'd rather be in there with them than be in here with the drunken ass.

Then without warning, his eyes rolled back in his head, and he collapsed on my bed. Oh great, now what? What I wanted to do was drag his ass down three flights of stairs, banging his head on each stair, and throw him in the front lawn. But I did still care about his well-being and didn't want another police report on his record. What I did do was walk downstairs to see if there was anyone in the lobby, to scope out the situation in hopes Mindy and Jonathan could help me get rid of my intruder. But as I peeked in the foyer, our dorm monitor sat watching TV, and I knew there would be no way we could sneak past her carrying a body. CRAP.

I walked back up the stairs, contemplating my situation, and decided just to leave him there to sleep it off for the night and escort him downstairs before Ryan would come over. God, why was this happening to me?

Knock knock. I was trying to get Mindy's attention. I knew she said only for emergencies, but I really felt this was an emergency. *Knock knock.* "What?" she said, pulling the door quickly open.

"I need your help." I was frantically trying to get her to understand the situation unfolding in my room.

"Did Ryan spend the night?" she said with a smile on her face.

"No."

"Then who did I hear talking to you earlier?" she asked in sleepy confusion. Motioning to her to enter my room, she quickly pulled on a nightgown, and Jonathan quickly got up too, following her as well.

"OH SHHITT." She held the word out to make it sound just as bad as the situation was. "What the hell is he doing here?" she asked, giving me a look.

"I didn't invite him. He just showed up at the door, drunk as a skunk, and passed out on my bed. What am I going to do?"

"Well," she said, "I don't think he's going to bother you tonight, but I would leave a trash can by the side of the bed just in case he decides to hurl." Oh great, if he pukes, I'm going to be even more pissed. "What am I going to tell Ryan?" I said, looking for a concerned answer.

"Don't worry, he'll be gone before you see Ryan, and he will be, hopefully, out of your hair for good." Thinking that would be a good plan. "If you call security, you know you are going to get into trouble, and if we try to carry his drunk ass downstairs, we will all get into trouble. Just let him sleep it off, and talk to him in the morning when he's sober." She was right. I really didn't want anything bad to happen to him, and if he got another ticket on his record, he would be facing some serious consequences. I wasn't that cruel. He could sleep it off, and I would talk to him in the morning. We all went to bed, and I slept on my king-size bed as far away from him as possible. I loved Ryan, and I didn't want anything to get in the way of that. Besides, if I called him, would he really believe me?

Chapter 12

After a night from hell and barely getting a wink of sleep, I finally looked at the clock, and it was 6:30 a.m. *God, wake up you horse's ass.* I just wanted him out of my room. When I would finally doze off during the night, he would roll over to my side in the stupor he was in and try to make the moves. So I would get up, move to the other side, and pray he stayed over there. We repeated this routine at least three more times until I finally made a bed on the floor in Mindy's room. I'm sure it was a damper on their activities, but I really think they understood. Mindy was always there for me, and Jonathan was understanding as well.

"I'm sorry I ruined your evening, guys," I said, pulling myself off the floor.

"Don't worry about it," Mindy said, knowing that I really liked Ryan, and she would do anything to get my ex out of the picture.

I was hoping when I walked back into my room he would have realized that I was nowhere around and leave without making any more trouble, but there he was, sitting at my desk chair, staring at me with a look of disappointment on his face.

"There you are," he said, knowing that I couldn't have been far away because I had left my purse and other personal belongings on the table, except my phone. Why didn't I have my phone? I would have more time to get him out of my room, and Ryan would not be on his way here. God, when was he going to show up? *Please don't come yet. Please don't come yet.*

"Yeah . . . are you ready to leave now?" I said, hoping he would leave with his tail between his legs, realizing what an ass he had been.

"Can't we talk now? I'm sober . . . and we don't have any distractions." He was talking as if we had something to settle, and maybe we did, but this was not the time or place. Ryan would be here soon.

"This is really not a good time," I tried to explain with such anguish in my face. He had to inquire more about my morning's activities.

"Why not? Who in the hell will be here this early in the morning?"

"None of your damn business, but I am expecting someone this morning, and I really don't want him to see you here."

"What happened to us? We were so happy once." He was trying to continue to work out whatever problem he seemed to want to conquer, but I wasn't having any of it.

"Listen, Gordon, you will always be my first love, and no one could ever take that away, and I only want the best for you, but I'm ready to move on. I'm sorry." Trying to appease his diligence of interrogating me, I asked him if we could meet later today to discuss this matter, just so he would leave.

"Please, I'm begging you. I need you to leave, please," I said as tears ran down my face.

"You really like this guy, don't you?" he said, looking as though his ego had been deflated beyond measure.

"Yes!" I had finally met a man that made me feel beyond loved. I know I barely knew him, but from the first day we met, all the ties that had bonded me to Gordon had slowly dissolved. I had tried to date other guys but always found myself drawn back into a relationship with Gordon, thinking there was no one else for me. But here I was, ready to snip every tie we had from the past and not think twice about it. "I care so much for him . . . I'm sorry, but I want a future with him, NOT with you. Can you understand?" I said, sitting there, hoping it soaked into his thick skull.

"You really don't love me anymore?" He was looking at me as though his chest were being crushed. Oh goodness, it was hard to see him that way. I did love him before, and I really didn't want anything bad happening to him, but this had to be it. "Did you ever love me?" he said, trying to find some string of hope to hang on to.

"Yes, I did, and you will always have a special place in my heart, but that was then, and this is now . . . So please leave," I said, hoping Ryan would not be pulling up soon.

"Fine. I'm out of here!" He said, grabbing his belongings and storming out the door. Thank goodness. Oh NO. A '66 Ford truck makes a definite sound when you hear it. I looked out the window, and yes, he was here. No. *Gordon, get out, please, before he sees you. Please.* He was getting closer, walking up the stairs of the dorm. I tried to hurry down the hallway as quickly as I could just in case they met each other and I had to explain the situation. *Feet, don't fail me now.* One more flight of stairs, and I was in the foyer. NO. They stood facing each other. Ryan looked in the doorway. Ryan looked at me. My feet wouldn't move. Move. What was Ryan thinking? They were standing by Ryan's truck now, and I didn't know what to do. What was he saying? Gordon walked off with a puffed up swagger, and Ryan looked at me again, turned swiftly around, and drove off without turning back.

Oh my god, what did Ryan think happened? As I watched Gordon drive out of the parking lot with a smug look on his face I shouted, "What did you do?"

Chapter 13

I ran up the stairs with rivers of tears flowing from my eyes. No . . . why didn't he talk to me? What did he think happened? And what did he tell him? I kept running. Running to the third floor felt like a marathon, but as I burst through the door and threw myself on the bed, crying uncontrollably, my body went numb.

"What did he do to you?" Mindy came running around the corner with a most concerned look. Tears were completely staining my pillow.

"Ryan knows Gordon was here," I said between sniffles and tears. "I don't know what to do. I must go to him and explain everything to him." I grabbed my keys and headed for the car.

How could I explain myself to him? What was I going to say? Would he believe me? I didn't know, but I had to try. I loved him; I hadn't said it yet, but I knew deep down I did. We shared such a wonderful night together, and surely, he would believe me . . . What was he thinking?

I pulled up in the driveway, and he met me outside the house with my phone in his hand.

I jumped out of the car with the hope he would be greeting me with open arms but knew by the look on his face I would be facing a challenge. I had never seen such a look of disappointment and betrayal. "Please let me explain . . ." I said in desperation as we get closer.

"Don't bother. I am so tired of putting my heart on the line and watching selfish people like you trample my trust."

"But wait—" I said in desperation.

"No. I am tired of being the pawn in this game . . . He told me everything I needed to hear, and I want you to leave." Hearing him say this made my heart feel like it was being crushed. How could he believe him, and how bad had he been hurt in the past? Obviously, pretty bad.

"NO . . . I can explain," I said with tears streaming down my face.

"It's not going to work . . . Last night was fun, but you need to find someone else," he said as he slammed the door to his house, and I heard the lock click.

"It wasn't what you think," I screamed, hoping he was listening. I sat there for a few moments, and then I heard the roar of the drums begin. He was playing with such passion and was doing it because he didn't want to hear me explain myself. *Oh, please stop . . . Please . . . I love you,* I thought, as the drums continued their thunder of pain.

What did he think Gordon and I had done? Will I ever get the chance to explain myself? I remembered I had the phone in my hand, so I began to text.

> Text: I need to talk to you. It's not what you thought.
> Please don't believe anything Gordon said.

I briefly heard the drums stop. He got it.

Reply: I'm done. Good-bye.

Text: Please . . . . nothing happened . . . I promise . . . .

Reply: I've heard that all before.

He wasn't going to believe me. Why? I picked up the phone again and texted the person who created this horrific mess.

Text: . . . . I hate you and never want to see you again . . . . Gordon . . . . you have ruined my life!

He didn't reply, probably knowing that he had caused the damage that he needed.

I went back to my dorm, barely able to drive because I was crying extremely hard I couldn't see the road. What could I do? Last night was the best night of my life. I didn't want to lose him.

Mindy met me at the door, not knowing what to see, and she observed that, obviously, the problem had not yet been fixed.

"He doesn't believe me . . ." I told her.

Chapter 14

I roamed through the halls in a trance for the next few days, hoping summer break would get here soon so I wouldn't have to avoid seeing him and seeing his eyes of disappointment. Where had he been? I hadn't seen him at band practice and wondered what had happened to him.

I drove by his house a few times in hopes I would see him outside and we could talk, but I never saw him. Where was he? I knew he might not want to talk, but I had to know that he was OK.

He might not care for me anymore, but I didn't want anything to ever happen to him.

Text: Deb . . . we need to talk

Oh, thank goodness. He wanted to talk. I could tell him that I was so sorry about what happened. My heart inflated just a little in hopes that we could work this all out and we could put this all behind us.

Reply: I agree . . . . we do need to talk . . . I'm sorry

Text: Be here at 5:00 . . . . we won't have a lot of
time . . . . but need to clear the air.

Man, he sounded pissed, and I was really not sure I could take this. I'd already spent three years of my life involved in a relationship where I felt I was always apologizing. I thought it was going to be different this time. Should I go just to hear what an untrustworthy person I was? "We won't have a lot of time." Why? Had he already moved on and had a date? Surely not. *Quit second-guessing the outcome.* I had been the worst about finding the worst in every situation.

Reply: I will be there!

Wait a minute; I didn't do anything wrong. Why am I feeling like the bad guy here? I did my best in the situation I was dealing with. I didn't sleep with anyone. I didn't kiss anyone. I didn't even sleep in the same room. Now I'm getting pissed. Why am I trying to defend that fact that he doesn't believe me? Why should I go? Is he the kind of person I want to spend my life with? God, help me make the right choice.

It was now two o'clock. I was sitting in my dorm, debating my future and whether I had one with Ryan. Remembering the wonderful evening we had together and how, in such a short time, I had found myself thinking about him.

I looked on the dresser and spied the little stuffed chick he placed in my car with the note that said, "To my favorite CHICK." We were compatible. We talked, and we could be so much more.

I was tired of playing games in relationships. I wanted someone who trusted me, who desired me, who loved me for who I am.

It was now four, so I decided to take a shower and hope for the best this afternoon. I hadn't seen Mindy all day, and I wondered where she'd been. I could have really used a friend this afternoon. She was probably with Jonathan, doing their thing, but I needed to talk to someone, and she usually gave pretty sound advice.

As I soaked in the shower, I was reminded of that beautiful night when we shared ourselves so freely. His touch reached inside my soul and made me feel wanted, desirable, and above all, loved, although he never said the words. Who said they loved each other after a few weeks of dating? Who? I guess it was only me. I desired his hands to be on me again. His lips to caress my body in any way he desired.

Four fifty was here, and I guessed I had better go. I was dressed in a very casual sundress with sandals. It was a beautiful night. He was standing by his truck. *Wait*, I thought, *I was supposed to meet him at his house. What's going on?* I walked up to him, ready to hear what he had to say, and by the look on his face, I was not sure of his mood.

Once again he was wearing his Wrangler jeans, boots, and cowboy hat—damn, he has a nice ass. *Stay focused on what's happening, Deb*, I told myself, ready for the worst but hoping for the best.

"Hello" was all I could say, not knowing what was fixing to happen. "I've missed you," I said, trying to lighten the haze I felt surrounding us like fog.

"Please get in the truck," he said as he opened the door for me, closing it with a start as soon as my leg went inside. He didn't look at me or anything. And where was he taking me? Did I trust him, or was he about to take me somewhere and give me a flogging away from his parents' house, away from the dorms. Where?

"Where are we going?" I asked, trying to get him to open up to me.

"I need you to be quiet until we get to our destination, please," he said, making me think that it might take awhile, and I was not good at staying quiet. This was so difficult.

We began to drive to a remote dirt road about ten miles out of town. Oh my god, he was so mad at me he was going to leave me out here for the buzzards. *Oh, get a grip, you idiot. He's not that kind of a person, but what is going on?* He sat quietly as we finally reached our destination.

We pulled into a quaint pond set down in a small valley near what we called the Northwest Woods Co. It was beautiful, and as we got closer, I noticed a light ahead. Four or five glimmering candles were lighting up what looked like a picnic area. "Where are we?" I asked, still trying to figure out what was going on.

"Shhhh" was all I got from him. "Be patient. I promise I will explain," he said calmly.

As we pulled up, he stopped just shy of the water and came around to open the door for me. I was almost afraid to leave the truck, but when he smiled at me, I knew there was no danger here, but I was still confused. Was he no longer mad at me? What happened that all of a sudden his feelings had changed? Or worse yet, he was going to throw me in the pond. *Get a grip, Deb.*

"Come with me," he said with a now gentle and reserved voice. I knew he still didn't want me to talk, so I did my best to keep my mouth closed. Truly, this was difficult.

We walked toward the glowing lights in the close distance. There, lying on the ground, was a blanket, a basket, and a thermos of Mickey's, our favorite beer. I was kind of giggling, knowing just how country he is. How wonderful. He had brought me here for a picnic, but wait, we still needed to talk. How could he have changed he mind so quick without me explaining everything to him?

He looked so handsome, and as I walked with him, he grabbed my hand and gently asked me to sit on the blanket. He smelled heavenly. Whatever cologne he wore, I liked it. I could tell he was nervous, but so was I. All I wanted to do was hold him until time stood still, but I knew he had something he wanted to say to me, and I needed to hear it.

He began to talk. "First of all . . . I'm sorry. I know when you looked at me the morning I came to see you, you didn't see trust in my eyes but blame and hatred, and for that, I am truly sorry. You tried to talk to me at my house, and I slammed the door in your face. I'm sorry. Since the first day I met you, I knew you were different, and

I wanted to believe that this time it was different. I have been hurt so many times I find it hard to open my heart to just anyone, but I knew you were different. Mindy told me everything and how you tried to get him to leave and how you slept on the floor in her room." I loved Mindy. She was my dearest friend, and now I know where she was all day. "I just couldn't bear the thought of anyone touching you except me. Will you forgive me?"

I flung my arms around him as tears of joy streamed down my face. Oh, thank goodness. I thought I had lost him forever. "I'm so sorry too . . . and of course, I forgive you."

This was never about sex; it was about trust, so we lay there on the blanket, holding each other. It felt so good to be with him again. All was right in the world, and I was a part of his life. Nothing could be perfect.

We ate the meal he had: fried chicken, mashed potatoes, corn, and rolls. So what if it said KFC on the box? He brought it, and it was special. He spooned the mashed potatoes into my mouth and smiled as if to say "Let's start over."

As he wrapped his arms around me, I softy said, "I love you," thinking he couldn't hear me. Within a few seconds, I heard a faint "I love you too." We fell asleep under the stars in each other's arms. It was beautiful.

Chapter 15

We woke with the beautiful Oklahoma sunrise, holding each other, remembering the evening before. "Do you really love me?" I said, hoping I would hear the same answer. His warm body felt so perfect next to mine. It was a chilly morning, but next to him, it was safe, it was warm, and it was all I'd ever wanted.

He was awakened by my question, nuzzled his nose into my hair, and told me, "More than you'll ever know." I never wanted to move. Why couldn't time just stop? I could handle a lifetime of this.

"What do you want to do today?" he asked as I could feel him pull me closer. As far as I was concerned, we could spend the whole day there under the covers, making love, but I wasn't sure what he had in mind, so I didn't bring it up. Last night wasn't about making love; it was about making up and trusting each other again. The closer I was to him, though, the more the thought of having him inside sounded enticing. I turned to face him, and as I did, I knew the answer to his question. I had never had sex in the middle of a field in the middle of the day. The most adventurous I had ever been was the fifty-yard line in high school, and that was pushing the envelope, but what the hell. I smiled my reassuring grin, hoping he would understand my intentions. His kiss was beyond soft, and as we entangled our bodies, I felt his intention with me as well. This wasn't about making up; it was about making out, and that was fine with me.

I thought to myself, *I must look like a sight.* But when he took my face in his hands, all the anxious feelings faded with the darkness of the morning light. He loved me for me. As he took me in his arms, he pulled me under him and slowly moved up and down my neck, placing soft kisses in specific areas as he moved across my body. Every muscle in my body ached with desire. I could feel the temperature in my body rising, and I knew I wanted this man. As I unbuttoned his shirt, I tangled my fingers on his chest. A soft moan came low from his throat as if he was feeling things he had never felt before. I can't imagine anyone ever hurting him, and I swore I would never do this to him. I pulled him down to my face and looked him in the eyes. "I love you . . . I've never felt like this before," I said, kissing him deeply as our tongues danced a slow dance together. And as he lifted me to him, I could tell he felt the same. We spent the morning making love, and if touching each other felt so right, I never wanted to be wrong again.

As he dropped me off at the dorm, being the gentleman that he was, he came and opened the door. I could feel people watching from the door, but I didn't care. He slipped his arm around me, making me feel like I was the only woman on the planet, and took me into his arms, leaned me up against the truck, and planted the most perfect kiss I had ever tasted. I swear I sucked all the air around me because it took my breath away. But when he Eskimo-kissed my nose, I had to giggle under his arms.

"Stop it. My friends are watching." I was acting as if I cared. Let them look because I want every single college girl to know he was MINE. *Keep looking, girls. See what I have.*

"Let them look. I only have eyes for you." He was smiling his sideways grin that once again melted me from head to toe. "Can I come over later?" he asked, knowing the answer would be yes.

"When? I might be washing my hair or something like that," I said with an even bigger grin. Knowing I was being a smart-ass, he flung me over his shoulder and walked up the stairs, deposited me at the dorm door, and said in front of everyone, "See you at seven." Then with his cowboy's nod of the head, he bid me adieu, and his sweet ass turned away and swaggered back to the truck. Damn, I was one lucky little shit.

Chapter 16

"Yep, that's mine!" I said as I walked through the gaping mouths of onlooking freshmen and sophomores. *Whores,* I thought to myself. *Don't even think about touching him,* I thought, *or you will pay the price.* I overheard one of them say "Damn!" I couldn't help but giggle under my breath.

I stepped in the door, and Mindy was standing there with a smile bigger than Texas. I couldn't help but run to her. "Thank you! Thank YOU! THANK YOU!" I said, hugging her uncontrollably. If it hadn't been for her, we might not be together.

"I take it you guys talked," she said as I let her breathe.

"How did you guess?" I said with a hint of sarcasm, giving her one more squeeze of thanks. "It was so wonderful . . ." And I began to tell her about the evening—and the morning too, of course. She sat there with intense eyes, smiling through the whole conversation, knowing it was because of her that this memory was even a part of my life now.

"So do you love him?" Mindy asked, knowing she already knew the answer as I said a brilliant "YES!" But how could this be? You don't fall in love with someone so easily. I had only known him for two weeks, and my life had been flipped upside down. He made me feel like every bad thing that had happened to me didn't matter . . . and it didn't at that moment.

"What about Gordon?" Mindy asked with reservation in her voice.

"What about him?" And just like that, I realized that I hadn't thought about Gordon for quite some time. Usually, thoughts of him surrounded my mind with every other guy I had dated, comparing what made him better than them, but NOT this time. I hadn't even thought about him, and I knew this was something special. All my thoughts were now focused on the one person who made me feel like a queen. There's no way I deserved this after the things I have done in my life.

I sat there thinking of the past and wondered why God would give me a break, remembering not so long ago, I was the one who thought she was pregnant and couldn't bear the thought of being pregnant in high school and jumped off the trampoline in hopes of a miscarriage. Apparently, it worked. There's no way God would forgive someone like me, allowing me the love I so desperately wanted my whole life.

Gordon had called one last time, and I hated to do it, but I was so mean to him. I was over him, and he needed to move on. I'm just glad I had never told him I was pregnant in school, or who knows what crazy drama we would still be in today. It's funny how things happen in your life for a reason and you really don't appreciate them until you look back on them and say, "Thank goodness for answered prayers." When you're young and stupid, you'd do just about anything for that person. Oh, I did. I knew Gordon would be OK. He was a good-looking guy, and someday he would find the right woman for him.

But trying to put those thoughts behind me, I tried to focus on the thought that, hopefully, Ryan would be calling soon. I cleaned up my room, knowing that tonight he might want to come to my room, and I didn't want him to know what I slob I really was. Mom was right; I do need a maid.

It was about seven o'clock, and I had just hopped out of the shower, shaved legs and all. He hadn't called yet, and I was beginning to worry. He had made it sound like it was a for-sure thing when he dropped me off in front of our crowd, but something must have come up. It was unusual for him not to call, and I began to worry. It was seven thirty, and I felt an uneasy feeling not really knowing why I was feeling this way. Seven forty-five, still no sign of Ryan, and I was praying it was a simple explanation, but no phone call, no text. I was worried.

Chapter 17

ing. "Oh, thank God," I said as I rushed to answer the phone.

"Hey, beautiful." Hearing his voice calmed me immediately.

"Where the hell have you been?" I was talking out loud again before I thought.

"Well, it's nice to hear your voice too," he said with a little malice, yet I could almost see a smile on his face through the phone lines.

"I'm sorry. I was just worried." I was thinking I sounded like a mother hen, and I was sure that was not what he wanted.

"I'll be there in thirty seconds." Without a good-bye, he was gone. In thirty seconds? Where the heck was he? I quickly looked out the front window of 321, and there was Izzy in all her glory.

And he wasn't kidding when he said thirty seconds. *Knock knock.* Wow. I'm really glad I cleaned my room. Hoping he didn't hear me run like a gazelle across my crowded dorm room, I flung the door open. Ready to pounce into his arms, I was taken aback by what I saw. Looking down, I saw a set of legs. But where his body should have been was a massive bouquet of roses. Oh my goodness, all I could do was cry. I had been given a flower once or twice in my life, but never an armful.

He brought them down so I could see his face, and all he could see were tears. Tears of joy, of course. "I hope you like them. I grew them especially for you." *Hahaha.* He beamed at me with that award-winning grin. All I wanted to do was rip them out of his arms and hold him close to me, but trying to be a little more grateful, I put them on my vanity by the window and stood back and admired his beautiful gesture. He was quite a romantic, something I really wasn't used to.

"Why?" I asked through a stream of tears, not really understanding that love was like this.

"Because I want you to know just how much you mean to me. And I want you to know that being with you makes me feel whole inside. I hate being away from you every second of the day and thought you would like them . . . Well, do you?"

"I love them," I said, swinging my arms around him, never wanting to let go. "These had to cost a fortune!" I was worrying again.

"Well, that was the problem for me being late. I took on another job so I could really spoil you," he said, smiling.

"Spoil away," I said, hoping he didn't think I was ungrateful. I couldn't help but feel the heat between us. He wanted me and only me. "Do you really love me?" I had to ask because this just didn't happen to me. I didn't deserve this.

"More than three words could ever express," he said, knowing what three words I had longed to hear from a perfect man, and here was my perfect man.

We had a fun evening going bowling, eating, and just enjoying each other. When we were at the bowling alley, a former friend, a baseball player, came up to me and gave me a hug. "Where the hell have you been, Deb? The parties haven't been the same without you."

Oh great, I had almost forgotten the fact that Ryan had saved me from a life of drunkenness. *Thanks for the reminder, Aaron.* "Well, I'd like to introduce you to my friend. This is Ryan," I said, noticing this burning look in his eyes. He was not happy.

"Nice to meet you, dude. So you're the one who stole her away." He was smiling like a fool.

"I guess so," he said as I could feel him tense like a board, standing next to me. When Ryan pulled me closer with almost a possessive touch, I could see in Aaron's eyes that he knew he had struck a nerve.

"Well, good luck, and maybe we'll see you around campus."

"Bye. Good luck next season," I said, trying to make light of our friendship.

"Thanks," he said as he joined his friends again.

"Well, that was odd," I said as I could still feel tenseness in the air. As I turned to look at Ryan, I could see he was upset. But why? He was just a friend, and we had done nothing together.

"I hate baseball," he said with a little shrug of his shoulders. Really, he's jealous, making me feel good in one hand and then bad in another.

"He's just a friend. I went and watched a few of their games this past year," I said, hoping he would see that he was only a friend.

"Where the hell is he from?" he asked, knowing that Aaron's accent gave that away easily.

"Boston." I was walking slowly to the concession bar, hoping he would drop the subject. "Are you really mad at me?" I said, hoping he wasn't this possessive, dominating creature . . . But then again, I like being submissive.

"I just don't want another man to even think of you in that way again," he said, lowering his voice.

"In what way?" I was acting like I was totally unaware of his rage.

Grabbing my arm, not harshly but with a mission, he quickly took me outside where our faithful Izzy was parked and stood me up against the door. It was dark enough outside that I really couldn't see his face, trying to predict his mood.

"I don't share well. I'm sure you've gathered that by now. But I can't stand that any other man has ever touched you, and as far as I am concerned, they never will again." Taking my mouth ravenously and holding me so close, I could tell this was going to end well. He was mine, and I was his. My protector, my lover, my all.

Chapter 18

School was almost out, and we were spending all the spare time we had together. My junior year of college was almost over, and it had been wonderful. Summer was quickly approaching, and I didn't want to go home to Seiling. I wanted to stay in Alva to be with Ryan but knew asking to move in with him was a no-no. Moms, they want you to play by the rules. Not like we didn't spend almost every night together, but anyway, I began looking for an apartment, hoping to find one cheap enough, but not a dump.

It would be nice to have a home of my own, and I was hoping that Mindy would like to move in too. She was from a small town too, and she and Jonathan were still hot and heavy. They were talking marriage, and I wasn't even close to that kind of commitment just yet, but I had to admit, it had crossed my mind once or twice.

I sat in the dorm room, looking through apartment ads, hoping to find a decent one. "Hey, Mindy!" I screamed across the suite room.

"Do you want to move to an apartment with me?" I was crossing my fingers, hoping she would agree.

"Really? Hell ya." And that was all I needed to hear as we sat on the bed together, contemplating which complexes would be the best. We finally picked one on Oklahoma Boulevard. It was on the second floor, but I didn't mind. I had been hauling things up dormitory stairs for three years, and I was used to it by now.

When I told Ryan about it, he was happy, but then I had the feeling he wasn't too. "What's up? You don't want me to get a place of my own and not have to worry about getting caught or signing in each time you come to visit me?" His look was puzzling.

"Will it be safe?" Here we go. My protector. I didn't mind the fact that he cared so much for me because I had never been the center of attention, usually just the girlfriend in the background. It was nice. I wasn't about to start complaining.

"Well, I'm sure there are locks on the door, and you can stay anytime you want to be my guard dog," I said with a smile.

"I'm serious. I've heard a lot about these apartments and how many girls have been hurt, and I just don't want you to be in any situation where anything could happen to you. You mean the world to me, and I told you I would always protect you." Shying away from my half smile. He did care, and I could tell by the way he looked and spoke with such concern and sincerity.

"Don't worry. If you're not here, I probably will be with you anyway," I said, smiling.

"Sounds good to me," he said as his shoulders lowered from relief.

We signed the contract the next day and began the time-consuming process of moving. It really didn't take that long since I didn't have anything major in the dorm room. We actually had to find a bed, sofa, refrigerator—you name it; we needed it. Mindy was extremely excited as well. Both Ryan and Jonathan helped us move in and started to make it look like a home.

It wasn't an oversized two-bedroom apartment. Small kitchen, decent living room, but no furniture. It looked huge. "Garage sales, here we come," said Mindy with a mission on her mind. The walls were painted the lovely hospital white, and we weren't allowed to paint them either, but it was home for now. Ryan still didn't like the idea of moving to an apartment where there wasn't much security.

As we made our final journey up the stairs, one of the bottom apartment doors flung open. "Hi, my name is Donald." He was reaching out a hand to me, welcoming me to the neighborhood. I could tell immediately Ryan didn't like him. Ryan introduced himself first, causing Donald to break eye contact with me, which did feel really strange.

"My name is Ryan, and this is Deb and Mindy." He was making us feel as though we weren't capable of introducing ourselves, but I knew exactly what he was doing. We were in the middle of a pissing contest, and Ryan was winning. Marking his territory like a wild animal. I gave him the glance of "You have nothing to worry about." Donald wasn't exactly a looker, but he did have what I thought was a pleasant personality. As soon as we made it up the stairs, Ryan made no effort in hushing his voice as he told me he never wanted me near him again.

"Don't let him in your apartment. Don't let him call. I don't trust him at all." Really. It was our first day, and we were already fighting with the neighbor. I reassured him that he had nothing to worry about.

"I'm not that stupid!" But unfortunately, he knew me all too well at this point in our relationship and knew I wasn't a very good judge of character. Donald seemed like a harmless fly to me.

We had finished unpacking all the items we had, and wow, did it look bare. One lazy boy, a small TV on a stand, and a bookshelf in the corner. We were quite the Betty Homemakers. We looked in the paper and saw that there were at least ten sales this Saturday, so we began to pool our funds to see just how much we had to spend on furnishings.

For heaven's sake, we didn't even have plates. Ryan looked around, wondering what we had gotten ourselves into. He began checking the locks on the windows and doors and discovered the window in Mindy's room had nothing but a stick in it to keep it from opening. "Oh, that's safe," he said, looking at me with a desperate look of "Let's find somewhere else."

We were on the second floor, for crying out loud. Who was going to shimmy up the side of the building? I simply told him, "As long as the stick is there, we are good to go." He didn't seem to think so. I walked into my room with the mattresses on the floor, wondering if I could find a frame for these quickly. After Ryan's thorough rundown of the place, he sauntered into the room, snuck up behind me, and in no particular way, whispered, "You do know we will have to anoint this room as well." He was kissing my hair.

"I can't wait," I said, turning to face him.

"I would rather you stayed at my folks' house upstairs than live here. I could keep you safe there."

"I'm a big girl," I said, pulling him to me to thank him for the gesture.

"OK . . . but I still look forward to our time here alone." He was giving me the sexiest desirable look. My face flushed, and I honestly couldn't wait.

When Mindy and I returned with our garage sale stash, I went to open the door, and it was unlocked. "Did you forget to lock the door?" I asked, hoping she would say yes, but she just looked bewildered. I took a quick look around and thought maybe we were just so excited about the move that we had just forgotten.

We liked the apartment after a while. Ryan was still worried, but I reassured him that everything would be OK. "Please let me ask my parents if you could stay upstairs at their house. I really don't like you staying there" was a repeated conversation we would have on many occasions.

"Have you seen your neighbor lately?" Ryan asked one morning. And come to think of it, I hadn't seen him much except once in a great while we would be coming in or going out at the same time. He seemed harmless, and actually, I overheard him having a conversation with another neighbor that he was majoring in law enforcement, so he couldn't be that bad. After I told Ryan about that, it still didn't seem to appease his feelings toward Donald.

Ryan was so protective. I loved it, but sometimes I felt like he didn't trust anyone. When he was over one afternoon, I happened to ask him why he felt so nervous around other people. "I'm just not a people person, and where you are concerned, I only want to keep you safe, and there are a lot of screwed-up people in this world." OK, I couldn't argue with that, but I was still too independent to let him rule all my decisions.

Mindy and I had decided we needed to celebrate our new home, so the plans for a party were in full swing. Yes, we had plenty of friends on campus and wanted to loosen up a little; we hadn't done that in months. I called Ryan to let him know what the plans were for Saturday, but he wasn't too keen on the whole idea. "Who will be there, and what is this for?" He was asking with the intent of intrusion.

"It's just some of our friends, and I promise it will be no big deal. Besides, you will be here to protect me, right?" I was hoping even though he hated crowds, he would attend in my behalf. I really didn't care if we had the party, but I wasn't going to let Mindy do this on her own. Besides, it was my apartment too.

"Well, I suppose I will have to be, right?" he said, making it sound like my bodyguard would be required to attend.

"I was hoping so. Besides, you might get lucky with some hot drunk chick. I hear she puts out when she's drunk." I was smiling uncontrollably.

"Yeah, that's what I heard too," he said, smiling devilishly.

Chapter 19

The date was set, the phone calls had been made, and we were ready to have some fun. Mindy was excited, and to be honest, I was too. I had missed hanging with some of my friends, but I would never admit that to Ryan. I didn't want him to think that I was nothing but miserable without him around, but to be honest, I usually was. I was glad he was coming even though I knew he would be checking out every person who walked through the door, making sure they were keeping their hands where they were supposed to. And I was surprised he didn't ask for IDs as they walked in the door. He actually kept his distance, keeping a watchful eye.

By 11:00 p.m., the party was in full swing, and the keg was half finished. Unfortunately, I had taken my fair share. "You better slow down," said Ryan with his look of concern. Here it was, just like the first date, I was being a stupid adolescent, and here he was, trying to keep me safe again. Whom was I kidding? I wanted him to keep me safe. There were a few people who had come that I really didn't know, but I thought, *Oh well, as long as they don't trash the place.*

There were also a few girls who showed up, and you could always tell the party trash girls. Their skirts were shorter than their IQs, and they hovered in packs. I thought in my drunken state, *Who the hell invited those wenches?* I kept an eye on them, making sure they kept their distance as I visited and enjoyed a few games of quarters. Ryan sat beside me most of the evening unless he felt pressured by the crowd, and occasionally, he would walk out on the patio to escape the horde of people. He wasn't much of a people person, and that was OK as long as he was into me.

Finishing a game, I glanced around but didn't see him. Apparently, he was outside again, so I decided to see how he was doing. To my surprise, I found him pinned in a corner, with wench number 1 and wench number 2 pawing at him. He didn't see me coming, and I could tell he was nervous just being around them. And I was not sure if it was the beer or just my sheer will of determination, but I grabbed the blond bimbo by the hair, yanked her off her high heels, and commenced to let her know she needed to get the fuck out of my house. Her face, along with Ryan's, was priceless. With a voice as low and soft so that only she could hear me, I looked her face-to-face and said, "Listen, bitch, if I ever see you even come close to my man again, I will rip your eyes out. Do you understand?"

She took a step back along with wench number 2 and headed for the door. Right then, I noticed Donald standing in my living room. Who the hell invited him in? Without hesitation, I grabbed Ryan's arm with the same intensity he had earlier grabbed me that day at the bowling alley and pulled him into my room. His eyes were full of heat; mine were sharing the same full-on intensity. "No one will touch you," I said, knowing my possessive instincts were kicking in without realizing it.

Once again, not knowing if it was the booze or just courage, I pushed him up against the closet door and swore I would never let go of him for at least an hour. This wasn't just passion; this was lust. I can understand how he felt when he saw me with another man, because my gut wrenched just thinking about another girl touching him.

By one o'clock, the party had settled down, and most people were beginning to leave. Which was fine except for the fact that some of them needed rides home, and there was no way it was going to be me giving them a ride. Poor Ryan was asked by many drunken fools to help get them to their apartments across town or to another party where they would find rides from there. He was such a good man, and I told him I would be waiting for him when he returned.

I was so tired. The house was a mess, but I didn't care. Mindy had told me earlier that she was leaving with Jonathan and that they might be back later, depending on what mood she was in. Mindy, you never knew what kind of mood she was in. So after looking at the mess, I decided that tomorrow would be a much better day to clean. As I walked to my bedroom, I noticed that Mindy's door was open, so I glanced in just to make sure there was no one there. I did notice the stick from her window was standing up next to the bed but didn't think anything of it. I was so tired and drunk. I fell into bed. Ryan had a key, so I wasn't worried about him getting back into the apartment, and I found myself drifting quickly.

Suddenly, I heard something crash in the other room. I didn't know how long I had been asleep but figured it was Ryan coming back from his taxi service. It sounded like books falling off a shelf. I'm sure he had tripped over something left in the wake of the party, so I just lay there, waiting for his warm body to wrap around mine. But he never came in. What was that, then, if it wasn't him? I was almost afraid to get out of the bed but knew it couldn't be anything wrong. Plus I was in the mood to take on the world after that tramp tried to take my man.

I gathered myself out of the bed and slowly opened the door to my room. The door made this awful sound that should come right out of a horror movie. Nothing a little WD-40 couldn't fix. But anyway, still not feeling scared, I happened to see a figure standing in the bathroom, and I could tell he was naked. I thought to myself, *If this was Ryan, he would already be in my room.* And then I noticed Mindy's door was open again, so it had to be Jonathan. Oh shit. I tried to be as casual as possible as I closed the door, pretending not to see him. Oh, that was a close one. I almost felt embarrassed until I realized, it was my door opening again. Why the hell was he coming in my room? I didn't want to turn around to keep from a very embarrassing moment but then I thought, *Ryan, you little devil you.* When I turned to see Donald standing buck naked, my heart sank to the floor. What was he doing here, and why was he naked? Dear god, why was he naked? I had always heard of rape victims fighting off their attackers but never thought I would be the one doing the fighting. And without thinking, I said, "Get the hell out of my house!" Without a second's notice, he came after me. Where was Ryan? Where was Ryan? I screamed, but he had me turned around so quickly and a hand over my mouth before I could do much more. *You are stronger than this*, I said to myself. *Fight. Fight. FIGHT.* Where the hell was Ryan? He should be here. I screamed again, somehow removing his hand from my mouth. He smelled of liquor and body odor. *God help me. Ryan, where are you?*

I could feel his clammy skin against mine, and it made me want to throw up. Then, as large as he was, he pulled me to him and once again put his hand over my mouth. "Stop screaming!" he said, pulling me tighter to his body. His breath was of bourbon and reeked as he said the words behind my ear. He pulled my hair to let me know he was in charge. The thought occurred to me that he had police training and knew all the moves to restrain someone. How in the hell could someone with police training be doing this to me?

"Leave me alone!" I said as I elbowed him in the ribs. A moan came from his throat, but it wasn't enough to make him release me.

"If you stop screaming, I will let you go," he said, and I thought, *What harm can it do?* So I stopped struggling. His body was ripped, and there was no way I was getting out of this unless I talked to him, trying to subdue whatever anger he was holding in.

The liquor was doing the talking. By this point, I was crying and couldn't help but scream again. "Get out of my fucking house!" As his arm came around to hit me, I closed my eyes, knowing what was coming, and within seconds, I saw him—my protector, my love—fly into the room and tackle Donald where he stood. Ryan had told me once when we were getting to know each other that he had been lead tackler on the football team, and at this point, I believed him. I actually felt sorry for the son of a bitch. OK, not really. Donald was paying the price, and I was loving the fact that Ryan had subdued him in one punch.

I sat on the edge of the bed, blubbering uncontrollably, trying to figure out what had just happened. Did I create this mess by having the party? How did he get in the house, and why me? I had never given him any inclination of being attracted to him. He lay there like a wet rag, with Ryan panting, making sure the bastard was knocked out cold. And then he looked over at me.

"I'm sorry, I thought I locked the door . . ."

"This isn't your fault," he said. "The door was locked."

I looked at him with a confused look. I swear I didn't let him in this house. God, would he think I wanted this to happen? I cried even harder, and he took me in his arms. "This wasn't your fault," he was whispering into my ear as he picked up the phone and called 911.

After further investigation, they found that he had walked around a twelve-inch ledge around the outside of the apartment complex and snuck in Mindy's window from the outside. I had noticed the bar was removed but didn't even think about it. Apparently, sometime during the party, he had come in and removed the stick in hopes of returning later.

Thank God, Ryan was there. I can't even imagine what might have happened if he hadn't been there. There would have been no way I could have fought him off; 135 pounds versus 220—not happening.

It was still only 4:00 a.m. when the police finally left, and I couldn't sleep alone or even think about staying in this house by myself. Ryan was talking to the last officer as he looked over at me with my legs curled under me, I was sobbing into my robe.

"Thank you, Officer," he said as he shook his hand and left.

"Are you mad at me?" I said, thinking he would be pissed, knowing that he didn't want this party in the first place. Had I pushed my limits too far this time? Would he be tired of taking care of this helpless little girl who couldn't be controlled? He walked over to me and sat next to me, pulling me into his lap, holding me like a small child, which felt so good. Safe, warm, forgiving.

"No, I'm not mad at you. I'm just thankful I was here to save you from something I was afraid might happen." He had warned me, but I didn't listen. When was I ever going to grow up and realize he only wanted what was best for me?

He picked me up in his arms and carried me to the bedroom and wrapped the covers around both of us. "Please don't go," I said with a whimper.

"I'm not going anywhere. Now hush and go to sleep." Surprisingly, even after the rush of excitement, I felt safe again and fell asleep in his arms.

Chapter 20

We woke the next morning with a frenzy of questions from Mindy as she walked into the broken door. I hadn't heard it the night before, but apparently, Ryan had broken down the door instead of using the key. Hearing me scream, he felt there was no time. Mindy felt horrible, and immediately we both held each other, thanking God for the outcome of the storm the night before.

"Thank God you were here," she said to Ryan with an appreciative look. "Jesus, I can't even think about what could have happened . . . maniac."

"Yeah, I guess you can't judge a book by its cover, that's for sure." Donald wasn't bad looking, wasn't cute either, but I would never have thought he would do what he did. Ryan, on the other hand, never trusted him, and now I know why.

We heard he was charged with robbery and assault and was only given two years' probation and moved out of the apartments after the incident. CREEP. I was really kind of pissed he wasn't charged with more, but was willing to put this whole incident behind me and move on.

I really tried hard to stay out of trouble just to ease the mind of Ryan. He only wanted what was best for me, and I was always pushing the envelope. I wondered if that was always a reason he loved me, because he knew I needed him. I know I needed him.

About a month later, Ryan was spending so much time at work, and I hardly ever got to see him in person. *He isn't my personal bodyguard, and he sure isn't getting paid for this nonsense*, I thought to myself. Surely, it was just because he was working two jobs, and I appreciated the fact he was a hard worker. Most kids my age were bumming off their parents, and I knew Ryan had been raised better.

We had been dating for four months, and each day was better than the next, but where was this relationship going? Did I want more? Did he want more? Marriage was never something we contemplated together, but I knew someday, or at least hoped someday, we would discuss the future. We were just enjoying each other right now.

I had kept my nose clean and was staying out of trouble, which to my surprise, Ryan was extremely grateful for, he had told me. He wished he could be with me more, but there was something wrong, and I couldn't put my finger on it.

It was a beautiful summer morning, and I heard the phone ring. Mindy had grabbed it before I could get to the phone and had hung up before I could even ask who it was. She was looking at me with sad eyes, so I asked who it was.

"Ryan . . . he said he wants to talk to you this evening and wondered if you could meet him?" *Well, sure*, I thought to myself, *but why didn't he just talk to me?* By the look on her face, I could tell his tone was not a positive one.

"What else did he say?" I asked impatiently.

"He said he just wanted to spend some time with you and go somewhere special one last time."

One last time. Whoa, he can't mean *us* one last time. I had been so good, and I hadn't been in any trouble. I knew he had been busy, but we had been through so much together.

"He said he was taking you somewhere in Enid, so be ready by five." Oh shit, it was four fifteen already.

As I heard Isabel drive up at 4:55, I was ready and at the door, waiting. I wore a black dress to try and look seductive and charming, thinking that I had lost his desire for me.

"You look nice tonight." He was scoping me out from head to toe as he opened the door for me.

"Where are we going?" I asked, hoping I would get that award-winning smile again.

"Enid," to answer short. He seemed nervous. I asked if he was OK, and we didn't talk much on the drive, which seemed to take forever.

We pulled into a little restaurant kind of in the back, a hideaway area called Sneakers. Wow, it was secluded, and as I looked at the door, I read "Closing business. Last day July 20th." It was the eighteenth. Oh, that's what he meant by doing something for the last time.

"Did you know this was closing?" I asked, hoping this was what he meant on the phone to Mindy.

"Actually, yeah, I did, and I wanted you to come here with me for the last time before it closed." For the first time all night, I think I breathed without choking, and a deep sigh came from my throat.

"What's wrong?" he said, looking at me, concerned. I didn't want him to think I thought this was the end, and I was just waiting to hear the dreadful "Sorry, it's not you, it's me" speech. But without realizing it, a small tear of relief ran down my check. I commenced to tell him what Mindy had said, and a mischievous smile ran across his face. "Oh my . . . I never had any intentions of losing you," he said. "On the contrary, I had other plans for this evening."

With that whole misunderstanding out of the way, I was ready to enjoy the rest of the evening. He took me to the mall to go eat ice cream, and of all places, me wearing a black dress, we went to the car races. You could say I wasn't dressed appropriately. He was country, and well, I usually was, but tonight, we were not on the same page as far as wardrobe was concerned.

He sat on almost the front bleacher seat, where everyone around us had the beer mugs, Grit R Done T-shirts, and here we were. At least he had jeans on and a cowboy hat. I sat next to him like a sore thumb, thinking, *What the hell are we doing here?*

As we sat down, Ryan stood up and told me he knew the friend in the announcer's box and wanted to pay him a visit. Not thinking I would want to wander around in my high heels and tight black dress, receiving stares from every redneck in the stadium, I chose to stay where I was, watching insane men wreck their cars and watching—another left turn.

As Ryan came back down to see me, he had a grin as big as Dallas on his face. "Good visit?" I asked, knowing there was something funny he wasn't telling me, but I didn't want to pressure an answer.

"Oh yeah, great visit," he said, smiling. OK, what was up? I knew Ryan by now and knew he was up to something, but what at a redneck get-together?

This was actually my first time at the car races, and he was remembering his youth as they would come here on many occasions and enjoy the races. My family's idea of a good time was going to the river and handfishing. So I guess we were both rednecks in our own special way.

As we were talking, we overheard the announcements: who was racing what, who was sponsoring whom, and "Please can we have your attention in the front of the stadium. There is a young man with a cowboy hat who has something he would like to say."

Oh my goodness, what was going on? I began looking for a man in a cowboy hat and realized the only man in a cowboy hat was the seventy-year-old three aisles down and Ryan. I looked over at him, confused by what was happening, and once again, the announcer proclaimed, "Take it away, Ryan." Holy shit, he just said *Ryan*. I looked over at him, and his eyes were filled with so much love. He stood up in front of all the stands, with every eye on him, took a box out of his pocket, took his hat off, got down on one knee—oh my god, this can't be happening! I could hear the women around me gasping for air, and sniffles surrounded us. I couldn't breathe. The announcer finally says, "So, DEB, are you gonna marry him or not?" I was frozen, but somehow, my head began to move up and down, and tears ran down my face. He rose in time to catch me jumping into his arms as the entire crowd cheered for us both. It was the best moment of my life.

Chapter 21

September 12, 1992, was the day we had picked to become man and wife, and it was here so quickly. Ryan had actually asked my dad for my hand in marriage in August of last year, but we wanted to wait at least a year to give Mom enough time to help make the dresses. She was a wiz on the sewing machine. Of course, my parents' first inclination was that I was pregnant, until we told them a year from September. I think my parents both had heart attacks that day. What was even better was, when Ryan asked my dad's permission to marry me, his answer was "Well, hell, she never listens to me anyway." To this day, I still have to laugh at that. I was never sure if it was a yes or no.

So here we are again, on the best day of my life, waiting to marry the man of my dreams, remembering the past few years and thinking how far we had come. He loves me, and I love him; it can't be better than this. My father, a man of few words, takes my arm and begins to walk me down the aisle. People are sitting on hay bales—yeah, we're still country—and the wedding is in the side yard of my parents' home. There are tiki torches for candles, and of course, in Oklahoma, there was wind. There had to be at least three hundred people gathered to watch me marry that man. It is simple, cute, and only meant for us.

The lights twinkle through the trees as the sun sets, and the look in Ryan's eyes is nothing short of forever.

As the minister announces us man and wife, I think to myself, *I do believe in miracles.*

Introduction to Book 2

"For better or worse, in sickness and in health . . ." These would be the words to haunt me for quite some time. We wanted a family, but was it in the cards for us? I wanted to believe it but sometimes had a hard time accepting the fact that you didn't always get what you wanted.

My eyes won't open, but I can hear the sound of people all around me. I know I'm not dead because I can hear my mom and, of course, Ryan as he is telling everyone the surgery was a success. Why can't I open my eyes? I know where I am, and I begin to move my arm to feel my chest. A gasp echoes across the room, and I can hear my mother crying softly. "It's OK, Mom . . . I can't see you, but I know you are here." I honestly try to will my eyes open, but I can't. Was the surgery a success? I was hoping to hear an answer from someone. I feel someone standing next to me, and I reach my hand, hoping to find a touch from someone I love, and I do. "Ryan," I say in a soft whisper, "please tell me, is everything going to be OK?"

He kisses my hand gently. "Yes, you are going to be fine, sweetheart."

Chapter 1

We sped away in the car, knowing that the next week would be nothing but pure fun and excitement. I had just married a man who not only made me feel like a queen but was also helping me realize that I was worth every little blessing that came our way.

The car was loaded, and we were off. (I was still picking the rice out of my hair the next morning.) What a wonderful day. I looked over at my husband—oh wow, my husband—and his smile told me everything. "What are you thinking?" I asked, wondering where that evil little grin was coming from.

"Oh, just everything . . . and all the things I want to do to you this week." He was looking as handsome as ever in his Wrangler jeans and pink tux shirt. I scooted as close to him as possible without disturbing his driving skills. *Till death do us part*, I think to myself.

The first place we stayed was the beautiful Monkey Island resort on Grand Lake. It had three wings of rooms and wasn't as busy as I thought it would be. Apparently, we were there in the off season. The trees around the buildings were changing colors, and the brisk, cool air felt so good as we arrived. When we pulled up to the door, we were met with a smile and a young man who opened the door for me and took our luggage inside.

As we were checking in, the foyer was ordained with beautiful furniture and glass figurines. After a few clicks at the computer, the clerk responded with "Enjoy your stay, Mr. and Mrs. Seevers." It was the first time I had heard those words, and I was taken aback. Ryan just smiled as he held out his hand and repeated what the clerk had just said with a victorious smile. Wow, I never thought it would feel this strange yet comfortable to be called another name. I could get used to this, but I did regret that my name was no longer Gilchrist; I liked that name too. I had been a Gilchrist for twenty-two years, and it was going to take some getting used to.

We followed the bellboy as he took our luggage to the appropriate room. With the zap of the card, we were shown into the suite. It was beautiful. Out the front window, you could see the lake as boats roamed back and forth through the choppy water. And to the other side, you could see massive homes built along the shore. It was breathtaking. Ryan tipped the man and shut the door behind him and leaned against the door, staring at me.

"Well, Mrs. Seevers, what would you like to do first?" he said, looking at me without a smile but with heat-intensive eyes, knowing, or at least hoping, what my answer would be.

"Go fishing, I think!" I was trying to keep a straight face as he looked at me confused. Then realizing I was just kidding, he told me he wasn't waiting till the evening to consummate our marriage; it was going to happen right now.

"Come here," he demanded, and to my surprise, I responded without hesitation. What, now that I was his wife, did I become this submissive little wuss? But at that moment, I didn't care. I wanted him just as bad as he wanted me.

He pulled me next to him, and I could feel the heat from his body, and I could feel the heat in my body race up and down over every ounce of my being. He held my face in his hands, looked me in the eyes, and said, "I'm ready to make love to the new Mrs. Ryan Seevers."

His kisses felt like the first every time we touched. Invading my mouth, took his time. There was no need to rush; we had a lifetime to share each other. I couldn't imagine it being any better than at this very moment.

We spent two wonderful days at Shangri-La, lying in each other's arms, making love, and just holding each other as though it were the only thing we existed to do. I didn't mind this existence at all. "You know, we haven't used protection once," I said, looking at him with some concern but not a lot. He just smiled and said he had realized it. What did that mean? Was he already ready for a family, and was I? The next day, we were ready for our next destination.

We were headed to a secluded resort by a quaint little town of Grove. It reminded me so much of the Colorado vacations I would always take with my family—minus the mountain view. The town was filled with mom-and-pop stores that reeked of the antiquated memorabilia of a much simpler time.

Our cabin number was 3, and it sat along the beach of the lake. We looked forward to fishing off the dock, boating, and whatever else the week entailed. I knew what I wanted to do all week, and it had nothing to do with fish, boats, or even romantic walks on the beach. But that was all a part of the package. As we unloaded our luggage once again, he grabbed me in his arms and carried me into the rustic cabin. "I know this isn't our threshold, but I just wanted to practice," he said, stepping back in time in our new little getaway. "The luggage can wait!" he said, throwing me on the bed. I had seen intense expressions but not the ones he was giving me. Would it be like this every time he looked at me? In one fell swoop, I grabbed his shirt as buttons flew in every direction. I pulled him closer to me. He looked at me with a hint of a smile, knowing I had just ruined one of his favorite shirts. My body convulsed as every kiss he landed sent charges up and down my spine. Throwing my head back in complete submission, I simply let the whole experience happen. He was so massive, and all I could do was hold my breath, trying not to scream and scare the surrounding visitors. Why would this week have to end?

"Did you bring any protection?" I was acting as though I sounded concerned, but not really, which was almost humorous, considering we had finished and were lying next to each other.

We fumbled and put ourselves together, and thankfully, no one had messed with our belongings outside the cabin. We had even left the door to the car wide open. We were crazy in love, and it felt perfect.

We sat in the evening on the dock, watching the sun set and not really caring if the fish were biting at all, although I would rather they did if we did fish. Actually, we would have a contest on who would catch the most. Ryan usually won because I was too busy watching his butt and missing the bites on my line. I didn't want this to end. But reality was looming in the next few days, and we would be heading back to the fact that a life awaited us back in Alva.

On our last night, we took a ferryboat ride around the lake, admiring all the beautiful homes, and we could see Shangri-La in the distance and just smiled at each other as we both remembered our stay there just a few short days ago. We would definitely have to come back and visit.

Chapter 2

We pulled back in to Alva on Sunday at 8:00 p.m. We didn't want to get back any earlier than we had to. We were exhausted, but to tell you the truth, I would do it over and over again and not care how much energy it took to keep up with him. Just being around him made me blush. We pulled into OUR new home. I had been living there for a year because after the incident at the apartments, I swore them off for life and began looking for a new place.

It was an adobe-looking house with the Mexican motif. It was painted simple beige and was home—our home. It had two bedrooms and a basement, which was where Ryan spent most of his time. Not that he was in trouble, ha-ha, but he had his drum set down there and his therapy was drumming. I'm not sure if he needed therapy after our marriage, but he was down there a lot. It would almost make the pictures rattle off the walls every time, but I didn't care. When he would return from downstairs sweaty, it was all I could do to wait till he got out of the shower.

But it was our home, and we loved it. Ryan worked as a jailer at the sheriff's office, and I worked as a waitress at a local steakhouse and was still at student at NWOSU there in Alva. We weren't too excited about getting back to the reality of life but knew it was inevitable.

For the next few weeks, all seemed normal, and life was great. We continued to have awesome sex, and apparently, we weren't worried about having a family because having protection never became an issue. But was I ready for this? Could I be a mom? I was going to school to be a teacher. Surely, if I thought I could handle them at school, I could manage a family. This was all moving way too quickly.

One night as we were lying together, I asked Ryan, "Are you ready to be a dad?" He would make a great dad. I had seen him with his little nephew.

"Well . . ." He was taking a breath to really think about the situation, "I really don't know. I think I would be a good dad, but I'm not ready to share you just yet." He was grabbing me closer to him. I could totally understand that, but deep down, I really wanted to make a little person with him. Little person—that's funny.

"If he or she was like either one of us, we'd be in trouble." With a grin, he said it. And he did have a point. You know the curse every parent puts on their child about having children who act just like you do? Well, I know it's a fact. And I'm sure my mom, just like every mom in the world, put that curse on me.

I wasn't a bad kid; I just liked to push the envelope, and well, what kid doesn't? As a teenager, I really found my barriers and wished I'd been a little less provocative and little more conservative as a young woman. I once thought I was pregnant in high school, and that really tarnished my relationship with my mom, and it took a long time for her to trust me again. I totally understood that. So was I ready to face a child like that? I was not sure.

We went to work the next morning, beginning normalcy again. Ryan, to the office, and I didn't have to leave until eleven for the lunch run. I didn't mind being a waitress, but many times, you had handsy old men in there whom you really just wanted to avoid but couldn't.

A few weeks went by, and I started to notice as I would go to work, the more I smelled the food, the more nauseated I would get. I didn't think they were cooking anything different, but my stomach would really get upset. I knew there were people getting the flu all over town, so I chalked it up to the flu and decided to stay home for a few days, trying to get rid of the awful feeling.

Ryan came home that night, asking what was wrong, and I just told him it was the flu, but he didn't think so. I couldn't keep anything down like the flu, but I didn't have a fever. I thought, *Great, my thyroid is messing up again.* I had been diagnosed with some weird disease, and it often made me feel tired and nauseated. I hated going to the doctor, but maybe it was that.

When I woke up the next day and I still felt lousy, I made an appointment with the doc for later that morning. Ryan ended up staying at home that day, so he went with me, thinking I might be too sick to drive myself back home. He hated to see me the way I was, and I hated feeling this way. For one thing, it was getting in the way of our extracurricular activities, and I really didn't like that at all, and something deep down told me it was something worse than what we were thinking. It's funny when your own body communicates with you and you don't even realize it.

We walked into the office, filled out all the proper paperwork, and as usual, sat around for an hour, waiting for that five-minute consultation with the doc. And like usual, they did all the proper previsit checklist, and this time, they even had me give a urine specimen. I only did that when I thought I had a kidney infection. Great, I hated kidney infections. I was never good at drinking water.

We sat in the waiting room, which seemed like forever, when the doc came in with a grin.

I thought to myself, *Either he's having a really great day or he just heard something really funny.* But what he had for me, I would never be ready for.

"Congratulations!" *Oh shit,* I thought. Ryan's face turned ash, and we weren't ready for this. We had only been married for a few short months, and we were not ready for this kind of news. "I hope you're ready to be parents!" he said with a smile.

"Me too?" I said, not quite ready to respond to his excitement.

I was excited, but we had just been married, and I wanted to spend more one on one with Ryan before the diapers, rash ointment, bottles, and three o'clock feedings began.

The doctor said he wanted to see me in the next two weeks to check on the progress. I knew we should have been using something. Ryan just sat there, not saying a word until we finally got in the car. "Well . . . I guess it could have been worse news!" I said with a morbid smile. He put his hand on my knee and squeezed.

"You'll make a great mom," he said with an even bigger grin.

We didn't know what to think about the whole situation, and we weren't sure of whom to tell. I'd always been told to wait a few months before announcing a baby's arrival just in case, but this was our first, and well, we were never thinking the worst.

I immediately called my mom. She was surprised, but not really. She was excited to have a grandchild and was just thankful I was married, considering our former mishaps in high school. We went on to tell his mom and dad, and they were a little more apprehensive, thinking it was way too soon. "Is that the way you like 'em, son, barefoot and pregnant?" Ha-ha, coming from a family of thirteen children.

"Hey, I like shoes, thank you very much," I told him, looking at him with a vindictive smile.

We were so excited, and the more we thought about it, the more I wanted to plan the baby's room, paint the house, and buy a minivan—OK, I couldn't do that. Ryan once told me, if we ever bought a minivan, he would shoot himself. I guess it must be a less manly thing to have. And I wasn't about to steal any of his manhood.

For the next few weeks, I continued to feel sick to my stomach, and the smell of anything strong just made me want to heave over and yack. But according to all the books, that was just the way it was with some women. Why did I have to be like all those women? I hated throwing up, and I had a hard time working around food. So I had to start looking for another job.

One morning in May, I woke up to very strenuous cramps, thinking it was just part of the whole pregnancy thing, but when I went to the bathroom, it became a reality that something was very wrong.

I immediately called Ryan, and he took me to the ER. Tears welled up in my eyes, and I felt like my insides were coming out; it hurt so badly. *Stop bleeding*, I kept telling my body. *Stop.* But it didn't listen to me. I lay there with my feet propped up, hoping I wasn't having a miscarriage.

They took a urine sample, x-rays, and blood tests as soon as I got in the door. I could tell the urgency as the nurses and doctors rushed around me, not saying a word.

The doctor came in after an hour or so and gave us a halfhearted smile. "I'm sorry, hun, but the urine test came back negative." Leaning over my lap, I grabbed my face with my hands and fell to pieces.

"I'm very sorry," he said to us both but was really directing it to Ryan. Ryan moved to where I was sitting and held me to his side. *What had happened?* I wondered. *Was it something I had done or could have avoided?* I felt like such a failure as a mother and as a woman.

We went home and tried to watch TV, but the whole house just fell silent.

Chapter 3

I know I hadn't been too far along, but it still hurt. Many women have miscarriages every day, but it doesn't mean we like that fact of life. Ryan held me close that evening, knowing I felt like a failure, and he wanted to reassure me that it wasn't anything I had done. It just wasn't in God's plan at that moment. He always knew what to say to make me feel better, but where was God in all this? Wasn't he on my side? I know I had screwed up in the past, but I was hoping for a little leniency.

Life went back to normal or as normal as I wanted to make it. After the miscarriage, I had become more determined to be a mom. I guess the incident really sparked a fire in my biological clock. I had the desire now, and there was no stopping me. Ryan was just going to have to lie there and pretend he enjoyed making a baby whether he wanted to or not.

Well, obviously, that wasn't going to work, but it sure was fun trying. For months we waited, practiced, waited, practiced, waited.

I went to the doctor a few times, thinking there was surely something wrong with me and a simple pill would fix our problems.

Once again, I went through a battery of tests, and other than my thyroid acting up, which I was already taking a pill for, there was nothing physically wrong with me.

So once again, we practiced and practiced, ha-ha. We didn't mind, really.

I would find myself, after every period, buying a pregnancy test, hoping for two lines this time. And every time, it would be just one. "Would you please stop trying so hard, hun?" Ryan told me on many occasions, hoping to get some kind of relief from my relentless badgering of "Lie there and pretend you like it" speech. I really think the pressure was getting to him. Well, I know it was getting to me too.

Why wasn't this happening for us? Every other couple in the world could have children, but we were having a hell of a time. It just didn't seem fair. Was God on my side anymore, and did he really care? The whole "Footprint" poem came to mind when I began thinking about all the rough times I was going through, and was he really carrying me, or was I alone in this?

Ryan struggled every day to help me cope with the fact that we weren't successful. "You know it will happen if you just stop trying!" My mom told me on many occasions. I just wanted a child. What was so hard about that? I would get so mad when I would go somewhere and find mothers who seemed to pop kids out left and right and not pay one bit of attention to them, and I couldn't even get a positive sign to show up on the magic stick. I was getting frustrated, beyond frustrated. When was it our turn for a miracle?

Well, that day came sooner than later. We had been married for about three years, and well, our lives were in the process of the everyday activities, so we enjoyed being together. We were still in our middle twenties, so I guess we had nothing to worry about.

Then came the day when the + finally appeared on the little stick, and I just about fainted in the bathroom, but instead, I screamed with joy. Ryan came running, hoping I hadn't fallen on my head or something. I smiled, and he knew immediately what was fixing to happen. I jumped into his arms and about knocked him over right there in the bathroom. "I knew it would happen," he said with a fair-weathered grin. I knew he was glad to no longer being my sex slave. I doubt if he really minded, but now it was all better.

I began my vitamin rituals each morning, and of course, the doctor told me to take it easy for the first few months just in case. I did quit my job at the restaurant and started working at the City of Alva. It was a nice sit-down job, and I wasn't on my feet, running around every day.

I was so excited about the future. We were going to have a little person together. It still cracked me up every time I thought about it. We had discussed, on many occasions, what it was going to be, and often, we had different opinions on what it was and what we were going to name our newest addition to the family. We knew we had to name them after his mother because everyone had always been named after his dad, Mallory, which, incidentally, is Ryan's first name. So we were thinking, if it was either a boy or girl, they would have the initials A. J. after his mother, Ada Janette.

I thought Ashtyn Trey would be a great name for a boy, wanting to name him after a young man who had died when I was in school, Trey Decker. He was the epitome of the all-American boy. Ryan told me that everyone would call him ashtray. Plus it wasn't an A. J. name. So we thought Ashtyn James. The James name had been in our family, and I thought it sounded good.

The girl's name was more difficult to figure out. I don't know why, but it never came to us, or at least, we didn't like the names we were finding. So we lay the idea to rest for a while, knowing we had plenty of time to figure it out.

A few weeks went by, and I felt fine, thinking the morning sickness would eventually catch up with my body, but it didn't. This wasn't unusual for some women that never had morning sickness.

Life was going along perfectly until we went in for our first ultrasound.

Ryan and I went in with the anticipation to hear a heartbeat that never came. "Where is he?" I asked the doc. And as we looked at the monitor, there was my little blip, but no heartbeat. My heart broke in two. "I'm sorry, Deb. There must be something wrong with the fetus," the doc said, trying to hide his desperation of finding any kind of heartbeat. Tears swelled in my eyes. I had failed Ryan again. He deserved someone who could give him a child, and it wasn't me.

We had to schedule a D and C operation, and as I rolled out into the recovery room, I saw Ryan's face. It was filled with so much love that I couldn't believe it. How could he love someone who couldn't give him a family? Wasn't that what life was all about? But as he stroked the tears away from my face, he gently said, "It will be OK, I promise." Would it? Could I hold the affections of a man for whom I couldn't be the woman I knew I should be? Would he still love me?

He never gave me any inclination that he was ever disappointed in me for not being able to conceive a child, but in my heart, I wanted to give him the world. I lay there in the hospital bed, bleeding, feeling empty and useless.

I didn't want to think about children anymore for a long time. I even had a hard time coping with the fact that Ryan still wanted to have sex, but I wasn't interested anymore. But unfortunately, I knew if I didn't, I would lose him completely. It wasn't that I didn't mind making love to the man who meant the world to me; it was just that I felt like a failure in this department.

I stopped trying to have children for a long time, and we, unfortunately, had two more miscarriages, and I had decided I had had enough. I couldn't go through another one. "I can't see you hurting like this anymore," said Ryan with a single tear running down his cheek. "I can't do anything to make it better, and your heart is breaking, and I can't fix it. I hate to see you hurting." Ryan was truly hurting too, and this was the only way he was coping with the situation as well. What were we doing wrong?

He told me after our last miscarriage that if we didn't have children by the age of thirty, we weren't going to try anymore. That made my heart sink, but in all reality, I knew it was the best for both of us. My heart and soul couldn't take it anymore. With my faith, I knew someday those four beautiful children would be waiting for me in heaven, and they would be perfect there. Thank God for faith. I was actually grateful at that point that I had a mom who made me go to church and drill the fact that God loved me no matter what was happening in my life.

My faith was my rock.

I was twenty-seven and Ryan, twenty-nine; our days of having children were quickly coming to an end.

Chapter 4

One day, I had been working at the church as their secretary, and a friend of mine had told me about a couple in the church who had adopted twin boys not too long ago. Wow. Adoption. Why didn't I think about that?

They were a very sweet couple, and I knew them, and so did Ryan. We sat one evening to ask them the process of adopting a child, and they filled us in on all the dos and don'ts of adopting.

"Is this what you want?" Ryan asked with reservation.

"I'm not sure. Do you want this?" I asked him, hoping for a glimmer of hope in his eyes.

"I just want you to be happy," he said, knowing that children were definitely a part of the wish list.

You know you always hear the horror stories about adoption, but then again, there are wonderful stories as well. My aunt and uncle had adopted two baby boys. They couldn't be happier, and especially since they were newborns, the whole adoption thing was even better. They wouldn't have to deal with a past and work through it. It would be Mommy and Daddy, and that was it.

But we did decide to put in our application. I didn't quite realize all the hoops you had to jump through just to adopt. It's amazing, like I said before, that any idiot could have children and could care less about them, but I had to get an anal cavity search to adopt one. OK, maybe I exaggerated a little about the anal search, but the truth was, they checked our bank account, which was usually overdrawn, and our savings, which had very little in it. And to top it all off, I had to write a paper explaining why we wanted children and how we would discipline our children. Really, I would discipline them the same way I was—with love and understanding and an occasional swat in the butt.

Wow, really. And one night, a man went to our home to inspect it, to make sure it was livable, I guess. We had two big dogs at the time and figured our chances would be slim to none anyway. But we went through with the whole process.

We turned our information in after Christmas in 1991 and waited, and waited, and practiced, and waited. It felt like life had come to a standstill and we were moving nowhere.

Working at the church really helped me focus my attentions on not what God hadn't provided for us but, rather, what he had given us.

Our love was the most important thing, and we began to share it with the Lord more and more. We both grew up in the church and knew what was right and what was wrong, but we had drifted. Our pastor, my boss, was great. He really helped me realize that life was one big blessing, and we just had to appreciate each precious gift he gives.

Once again, time was sneaking up on us, and Ryan's reminder crept into my thoughts once again. "If we don't have children before I'm thirty, we aren't going to." Did he really mean it? I had hoped not, but I was praying that a miracle would happen, and it did.

On almost exactly twelve months to the day we sent in our application, we were called, but we weren't home. "You've got to be kidding me," I said to Ryan, reaching for the phone as fast as I could to return the call. I wasn't even thinking, but it was a Saturday plus New Year's Eve Day, and there was no way anyone would be in the office that day, but you never know. So I left a message.

We listened to the answering machine, again and again, "Hello, my name is Roger Gossard, and I am an attorney in Coffeyville. I am happy to inform you that a mother has chosen you to be her child's parents. Please call me as soon as you get this message."

It almost felt unreal. Like we were in this crazy prank and someone was going to jump out from behind the couch and go "Just kidding." But oh, that would have been an awful joke.

The next day was church, and we were so excited to tell everyone that we would be getting a phone call hopefully soon about our soon-to-be little person. Our friends were so excited, and as I watched Ryan playing the drums, he beamed with anticipation. I took my phone into the church just in case but never thought in a million years he would call today.

"My Redeemer lives—" As I raised my hands to worship, someone grabbed my arms and yelled at me, "Your phone is ringing!" I grabbed it and ran out of the church, trying to get to a place where I could hear the person on the other line. And as I ran up the aisle, people were cheering and yelling praises as I darted out the door.

"Hello," I said with an airy voice. I didn't even look at the number. It could have been someone I knew, but at that moment, I didn't care.

"Yes . . . is this Debra Seevers?"

"Yes, it is," I tried to say with a calm voice.

"My name is Roger Gossard, and I was hoping to get a hold of you," he said with a sigh of relief.

"I am so sorry we missed your phone call the other day," I said, hoping we hadn't missed our chance of being parents.

"Well, it was New Year's Eve, and I was just taking a chance you might be at home," Roger replied. "Why, I called was because I have a young woman here who would like to meet you." He paused briefly.

"Really . . . is everything OK?" I asked, hoping she wouldn't change her mind after she saw us.

"No, not at all. She just wanted to meet the people she had picked before she agreed to allow you to adopt her newborn baby due in thirty days!" *Thirty days. Oh my goodness*, I thought to myself. Most moms have nine months to prepare for this. *Thirty days.*

"Wow, we would love to meet her. Just let us know where and when," I sighed with relief.

"Well, there is just one thing I need to know." *Oh no, here we go.* There was something she didn't like about our application. She had doubts about us as parents. What was it?

"The birth mother wanted to know if you cared if the child was of mixed race?" *What did he mean?* "The child will be half black. Would you care?" *Would I care? Are you kidding?* I thought to myself.

"I wouldn't care if she was chocolate, strawberry, or vanilla with sprinkles," I said, sincerely yet humorously commenting on his question.

"Well, all right then, I will let her know and get back with you on the date and time. Have a nice day, Mrs. Seevers, and we will be talking with you very soon."

"Thank you" was all I could get out of my mouth.

I stumbled back into the church as Ryan was finishing up playing the drums, and I ran into his arms, holding him so tight, not caring about what everyone else in the church thought. We were going to be parents. "Hi, Daddy," I said to break the news to him.

Chapter 5

The phone stayed stuck to my side as seconds and hours went by. We were so excited about what had happened that we hardly slept that evening. Ryan went to the sheriff's office, and I was working at the school at the time. We were on cloud nine, thinking of our future and what it would bring. We told everyone what was happening, and whenever the phone would ring, everyone listened until they would figure out it was Ryan or someone else they knew.

I was sitting in the school, helping with a reading class, when I got it.

"Hello, Mrs. Seevers, this is Roger Gossard. How are you?" he said

"Well, to be truthful, I haven't slept a wink since you called, and I can't wait to meet her. Do you have a time for us?" I said, talking anxiously.

"Yes, please be at my office at 450 Sycamore Street in Coffeyville at ten a.m. Thurs. morning. Can you make it then?"

"Oh, don't worry. We will be there," I said, almost busting my leg on the kiddie table that I was sitting on when I hung up the phone.

I ran down to the principal's office and told her what was happening, and she immediately gave me that day off, no questions asked.

We lay in the bed, thinking, not even talking. I had to thank God, and I rolled over and held Ryan. "I may not have been able to give you a child, but I promise to be the best mother I can," I said, with tears running down my cheeks.

"This child will be loved just the same," he said with a quiver on his chin. "I can't wait to meet her." With a smile.

"But what if it's a boy?" I said with an almost defiant smile.

"I don't care as long as IT is healthy." That was one thing we could agree upon. We fell asleep together, in each other's arms.

Thursday was here, and we were racing to Coffeyville—literally, I mean racing. He knew most cops between Alva and the interstate, and he was going to use every card he had if he needed to use them in case we got pulled over.

"So what are we going to name him or her?" I said, thinking we only had thirty days to figure this one out.

"Well . . . we still need to think of A. J. names," he said, knowing how much it would mean to his mom. And being the smart aleck that he is, he said, "Hey, let's call her Shaniqua." I about slapped him. Plus it wasn't an A. J. name. Goober. He just smiled at me to try to lighten the mood of the anxious cargo.

"How about Amberlee for the first name?" I said, knowing my sister's name was Amber, and it was an awesome name just like my sister.

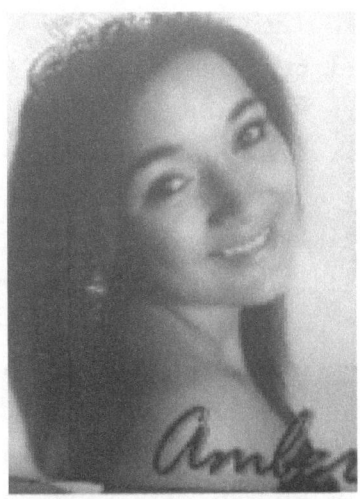

"Sounds good to me. Since I am using my mom's initials, we could use your sister's name." *But what for the*—and there it was. It just popped out of our mouths at the same time: JASMINE. Perfect. AMBERLEE JASMINE SEEVERS.

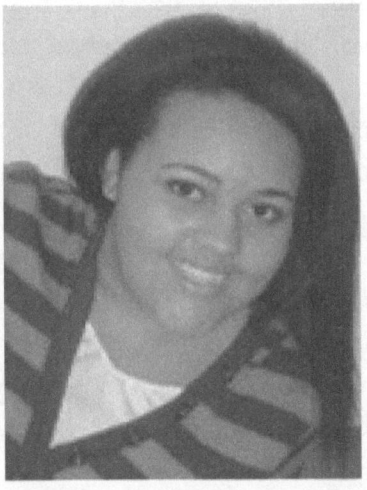

We pulled into the parking lot, and we both took a deep breath. Would we be what she wanted for her child? Would we fit the mold of whom she was looking for? God, I hoped we did.

Roger met us at the door. We were now on first-name basis, I guess. It seemed weird, but he always felt like family and treated us as though we were here. "Hello, Ryan and Deb. I'd like you to meet Tonya," he said as she smiled at us both, trying to gracefully get out of the chair and greet us both. She was definitely nine months pregnant and feeling it. I looked her in the face and realized we looked a lot alike. She was a bit taller than myself and Ryan but was as pale as me, and we had a lot of the same bone structures in our faces. She greeted us with a wonderful hug and smile. She didn't portray the typical mother who would be giving up her child for adoption. I was expecting this adolescent girl who regretted being there, not really wanting to be a part of this whole process but was being forced to do this, but she wasn't. Tonya was kind and seemed to have a true feeling of love for what she was doing. That really made me feel good about meeting her.

We sat and visited for at least an hour, and at one point, we had met her older daughter, and to our surprise, her name was Amber too. She was so beautiful. We told her, if her next child was as cute as Amber, we'd take two. She smiled with appreciation. Amber jumped into Ryan's lap and just started talking like they had been buds forever. It was so great to see him with her. It looked so natural, and he was loving the fact that she wanted to stay with him rather than sit on her own mommy's lap.

The longer we sat and visited, the more relaxed the situation became. Mr. Gossard went over all the legal aspects of the situation and let us know what we would be responsible for, and we sat there amazed at what we were a part of. We were going to be parents, and life was going to be change really quickly. "When is your baby due?" I asked, hoping to lighten the mood.

"January thirty-first," Tonya said with a smile. I couldn't believe it; it was my birthday too.

This couldn't be more perfect than if I had scripted it in a book.

As we drove home, we were almost in a complete fog of complete serenity and happiness. "We have twenty-seven days to get things figured out," I said as I looked over at Ryan with wide eyes.

"Yeah . . . I guess you are getting an amazing birthday present this year. Good thing I didn't buy you anything yet. It would pale in comparison." Ha-ha. He was smiling sweetly. He was right about that.

There was so much to do. We needed a crib, car seat, bottles, diapers, clothes—oh my goodness, we needed everything. We also had a house of love so ready for this little surprise. What would they care about as long as there was love? And there was plenty of that to go around.

The next few weeks were filled with anxious grandparents wondering what they could do to help us prepare for what was sure to be the ride of our lives.

Chapter 6

When we had first heard about how the child would be of mixed race, we really didn't care, but as we thought about our families, we truly wondered if it would be an issue with them.

We didn't care what this child looked like, but his family was from the Deep South, and well, where I grew up, there was only one family of African Americans, and well, we just didn't know what the reaction would be. And to be quite frank, we really didn't give a shit what anyone thought anyway.

This little person would be given everything we could possibly give. We knew we would be faced with the reality of prejudice but knew that we would handle it when it came. God was giving us a miracle, and nothing was about to stand in the way of our precious gift. And that was exactly what this was, a gift.

So all we had to do was wait. I was never very good at waiting.

We tried to go along with life as normal as possible, but it was really hard to keep from the reality of how life would be changing. As I sat in the teachers' lounge, the ladies would grill me each day, asking me when the baby was coming, and all I could say was on my birthday. They were just as excited for me as I was for myself. They informed me that I had to take the baby to the school as soon as possible. I promised.

"Hey, Deb?" coming from the secretary's office. "There's a phone call for you." Oh wow, who would be calling me at the school? I knew I had left that number for an emergency on my phone, but why didn't my phone work?

I pulled my phone out of my purse and realized that the battery was dead. Oh crap. In all the excitement, I had forgotten to plug it in to charge.

"Hello," I said, wondering who in the world was calling me.

"Yeah, Deb, this is Roger, and Tonya wanted me to let you know she has been induced this afternoon and wanted you and Ryan to be here for the birth." Oh my goodness, this was really happening.

"Thank you so much. We will be there as soon as we can," I said, almost hanging up on him in the excitement of the whole phone call.

"I need off, Lucy!" I said to the secretary with all the excitement of a five-year-old on Christmas morning.

"When?" she asked, sounding a little concerned.

"NOW! My baby is coming!" I said, almost shouting with hallelujahs.

"Oh my goodness," she said, grabbing me and giving me a tremendous hug.

The next thing I knew, I was throwing myself down the hallway in a full run as I heard over the speaker system, "If I could have your attention, we want to wish Mrs. Seevers a safe journey as she and her husband go and get their new baby this afternoon." You could hear cheers echoing down the hallway. Apparently, they were as excited as I was.

After we called our parents, we were driving wildly to Coffeyville, hoping to make it for the delivery. I was so excited to know Tonya wanted us there for the delivery. God, I hope we make it in time. My mom had informed me that she would be leaving ASAP to join us, but it was an even farther drive for her. Coffeyville was about a five-hour drive, and we didn't know how far along she was, so the anxiety of not knowing what was going on was killing us.

I knew it was February 3 and it was past her due date, but would her labor take as many hours as I have heard it could? I was actually glad she/he wasn't born on my birthday. I wanted their day to be just for him/her. I was really having a hard time not knowing what sex the baby was going to be, but deep down, I knew it was a baby boy. I don't know why; it was just how I felt.

"It's going to be a girl," Ryan said with confidence.

"Oh, how do you know?" I said, responding sarcastically with a grin. We had seen a sonogram of the baby, and well, I'm not a doctor, and I didn't know what I was looking for and neither did Ryan, but he was adamant it was a little girl. I really didn't care as long as they were healthy.

We screeched into the parking lot and made our way to the third floor of the hospital to find Roger waiting for us there. "Wow, I think you made it here in record time," he said with a smile.

"We promise we won't drive that fast going back," he said with a smile.

"Are you ready for all this, Dad?" I said, looking at Ryan.

"Well, I better be because it's really happening." He was sighing with relief, knowing that this was what we both wanted. "Yeah, and just in time," he said with a confident look, causing me to become confused.

"What do you mean?" I said, trying to figure out his intentions.

"My thirtieth birthday is in two months, remember?" he said, smiling with a victorious grin.

"Oh yeah," I said, thanking God for the wonderful timing. I never knew if he really meant giving up at thirty, but I wasn't about to argue with the joyous news coming soon.

Boy or girl?

We meekly walked into Tonya's room as she was dealing with labor pains, and we smiled, bringing her a bouquet of flowers to brighten up the mundane decorations of the hospital.

"How are you feeling?" I knew it was a stupid question, but I asked it anyways.

"Oh, with the epidural, I'm not feeling much," she said with a smile. "I'm so glad you could get here," she said with a very sincere grin.

"We wouldn't miss it for the world. We are just so blessed that you are giving us this opportunity." I was smiling.

"I couldn't ask for better people to have my child be a part of their lives."

We sat and visited about family and how she had struggled but had her church family to help her. I was glad to know she had been going to church. She told me about any health issues that her family may have had, in case we needed health information for future use, and calmly talked about how we should not worry about her changing her mind about coming back and taking the baby. To be honest, that was one of my worries. I would get attached and the mother would want the baby back. I had heard that so many times, and to hear her say that really helped ease my mind on that matter.

As I was talking with Tonya, Ryan was out in the lobby, discussing any legal matters we might need to deal with at this point. Roger had told Ryan that the biological father, who was a prominent business owner with a family, did not want to sign the papers. Roger, with his very good negotiating skills, persuaded him to sign or else he would have to ask his wife for permission. He ended up signing without any more worries. Roger was a guy who crossed all his t's and dotted all his i's. There were never any loose ends where he was concerned, and that helped us feel more comfortable in the situation.

Tonya had been in labor for over twelve hours, and we were beginning to worry about the progress. She hadn't dilated past a five for four hours, and we were at a standstill. OK, she was at a standstill. I was merely the bystander who felt so sorry for her at this point. She was beginning to feel the pain again, and I told her to squeeze my hand whenever she needed to.

Meanwhile, my mom showed up, and Ryan decided, since the process was taking a slow pace, to take my mom to find a motel room before it got any later. We weren't going to stay in the motel but rather be with the baby all night, but Mom didn't have anywhere to go, so off they went.

As I was coming back from visiting the bathroom, I heard the bustle of many people in Tonya's room. I peeked in to find the rush of doctors, nurses, and other personnel. Had something happened? Was everything OK? What was going on? I tried to get the attention of the nurses, but they simply had more on their mind than chatting with me. Finally realizing Tonya had dilated from a five to a nine in thirty minutes, it was time for her to push. Oh my goodness, where was Ryan for all this? He was going to miss it. NO. *Hurry, Ryan.* No. I decided to put the video camera in the window and turn it on just so he could have a visual of all that was going to happen. I didn't tell anyone what I had done, and to be honest, I don't think they really cared. I angled the camera just right to make sure it wasn't too detailed, if you know what I mean.

"PUSH," the doctor said, trying to get Tonya to focus on her mission.

"One, two, three, four, five, six, seven, eight, nine, ten—AHHHH!"

"PUSH. One, two, three . . ." I told her to hold my hand if she needed to hang on to something. I swear she about broke my hand, but I really didn't care. Where in the hell was Ryan?

As the doctor got the salad spoons—as I like to call them—I heard him say something about her head being stuck. Oh my goodness, that couldn't be good. *Please hurry. This is my baby you're talking about,* I said to myself. And in less than five minutes, I saw a head full of hair come peeking out. Wow, did she have hair! I think she came out with an Afro. As the doctor held our new baby girl in the air, tears swelled up in my eyes, and both Tonya and I began to cry.

"Do you want to cut the cord?" the doctor asked. Yes was all I could mutter out without sounding like a complete idiot. I was in heaven, and I was there, cutting the cord of our newborn baby girl. It was the most beautiful thing I had been a part of, and I was here to witness it. *Oh, Ryan, where are you?*

As they were cleaning her up, I heard the shuffle of people outside the door, trying to get in. It was Ryan, and he was getting ready to walk into the room when she was still on the table in stirrups.

"Whoa," I said, stopping him at the door. His face was ashen, and it looked like he was about to pass out.

"They told me when I got off the elevator that I was a dad," he said in a soft whisper.

"Yes, you are. And you were right . . . It's a baby girl . . . Amberlee Jasmine, meet your new daddy," I said, handing him the greatest gift we had ever received in our lives. He held her nervously, but like a new father smiling from ear to ear. Tears rolled down his cheeks as he kissed her forehead. It was another beautiful thing to see. Daddies always have a special place in their daughters' hearts. I know I do with my dad, and I was witnessing the birth of another wonderful daddy-daughter moment in life.

Chapter 7

She was the most beautiful child we had ever laid eyes on. After they took her away to do all the test of nine pounds, twelve ounces, and twenty-one inches long, we held her, staring at her glowing big brown eyes. "Hello, beautiful. So glad to finally meet you," I said as a tear rolled down my cheek as she cooed in my arms. I didn't know if I was ready to be a mother up to this point, but I knew I would do anything for this little person in my arms. It was amazing how color was never an issue, and even when I held her for the first time, I never saw color. We saw a bright-eyed daughter whom we looked forward to spoiling for the rest of her life.

My mom quietly came into the room as they had finished helping Tonya with her stitches. She had been crying. I had seen that face before. Apparently, she had been talking with our attorney and hearing all the chatter coming from the room. She held Jasmine in her arms, and there was such a connection. Her first granddaughter folded into her arms. Tears streamed down her cheek as she looked up at me and told me how beautiful she was.

We got to spend the first night of Jasmine's life with her in the hospital room. Ryan was also honored to change her first dirty diaper. "What is this, tar?" he said as it took ten wet wipes to clean off her little backside. The first diaper change is always very interesting. I always said, if we kept waste, we could naturally tar a roof or something useful. We really had no idea what we were doing. I was so glad to have Mom there to help us on our interesting path of parenthood.

As morning came, I stepped into Tonya's room to see how she was doing, and surprisingly, she was feeling better. I asked her if there was anything she would like, and she requested KFC food.

Immediately, Ryan jumped in the car and went and got it for her. We would do just about anything for this woman at this point. She was willing to give up a part of her life, something I don't even think I could have done, and if KFC was what she was craving, well, KFC it was.

Tonya came from a good church family, thank goodness, and we had been discussing having a baby dedication or ceremony in support of her adoption. Tonya had asked her pastor to go, and so did we, and they were glad to travel the five hours to get there.

The next morning, we held our little ceremony in the hospital. We all gathered as we told each other how much this meant to each of us, and as Tonya held Jasmine in her arms, the true sight of love was in the room. She was willing to give up her child to give her a life she knew she couldn't provide for her. She said her last farewell to Jasmine, or Nora Belle as she had named her, and handed her to me with tears running freely down both our faces. She hugged us as we all sang a hymn. Later we shared a steak dinner together that was set up by our attorney, and we enjoyed a wonderful meal together, making promises to each other.

"Please tell Jasmine that I love her and that I will never forget her," Tonya pleaded.

"Absolutely, I promise," I said, telling her sincerely that I would.

Tonya was not a bad person; she was just in a bad situation, and I knew she was sincere about what she was doing. We quietly said our good-byes, she gently kissed Jasmine on the forehead, and we parted ways.

We packed up Jasmine in the car seat and headed home. But we actually couldn't go home because of the State of Kansas. It was told to us we had to stay in the state for five days and not cross a border or it would be considered kidnapping. Wow, what rules. So we went to my grandparents in Kiowa and spent the week. Of course, my grandparents didn't mind. My grandfather was a doctor, and he gave Jasmine her first very thorough checkup. She actually got her first bath in my grandparents' sink that week. They really bonded that week. They loved being the first to really spoil her, and I was so glad they could have that opportunity.

We did cross the border a few times since Alva was only thirty miles away and Kiowa was only half a mile away from the Oklahoma border. We did call our attorney to make sure it was OK, just as a precaution. We didn't want to do anything that people would consider reckless. In the state of Kansas, the mother had thirty days to change her mind, and we didn't want to cause any strife or indecisions on the mother's part. After all, who would want someone raising their child if they couldn't follow simple instructions? So we were a good mom and dad, ha-ha.

Chapter 8

The next week, we were so excited about going home. Wow, home with our new baby. I was enjoying the fact that I didn't have to recover from stitches, labor pains, or all those great things from giving birth. I didn't care how I got a baby. I'm just glad I had this beautiful baby in my arms.

She was rather adorable, but I was a little biased. She had sun-touched skin and the curliest hair. I could put bows and ribbons in it from the first day we brought her home.

People from the church were so excited about having a shower for Jasmine. We were actually greeted by a beautifully decorated front yard that had "Welcome Home, Baby" balloons and signs all over, courtesy of our friends at the church in Hopeton.

We brought her into her room that Uncle John had just painted with bears and rabbits all over the walls. It still smelled of fresh paint, and Dad had put closets on each side of the wall to accommodate all the items she would need. The baby bed was neatly tucked into the corner, where her freshly washed blankets and sheets awaited to put the sleepy little babe on. Above the bed was a cute mobile that played "Rock-a-Bye, Baby" and spun cute characters that matched the bumper material along the bed.

Our life was perfect, and all the world within it was perfect too.

She actually slept through most of the nights and would wake up around five each morning. I sat up with her the first night, just holding her, hoping this wasn't the most wonderful dream I had ever had to wake up crying from, knowing it wasn't real. But this was our life, and holding Jasmine in my arms was so perfect. As she would fuss a little, all I simply had to do was rub over her eyebrows and softly touch her eyelids, gently, and she would be out like a light.

Watching Ryan with her was something of a miracle to see. Knowing that just a few short months ago he told me that if we didn't have kids before his birthday, we just wouldn't have any, and here he was, changing dirty diapers, warming bottles, and giving baths like a trooper. Actually, I had to fight him for the duties because he loved being a dad so much he wanted the honor most of the time. If you can call changing a green diaper an honor. Well, I didn't mind letting him, ha-ha.

Ryan had been given a week off to help us adjust to baby life, and I was very thankful. The school had given me eight weeks of maternity leave, and I was so glad to have that time with her. "It's your turn," I said as four o'clock came early a few mornings. But we were just getting ready for what was about to happen to our lives.

The baby showers were so wonderful. We got everything from twelve months' worth of clothing to a six-month supply of diapers, wipes, powder, and every ointment imaginable. She was completely spoiled.

Chapter 9

March couldn't come fast enough as we waited to have the final papers to show we were legally her mom and dad. But from the time she was born up to thirty days, she had that opportunity to change her mind. Each day when the phone would ring, I almost cringed the first few times but got used to it after a while. At first, it didn't bother me, but as the thirty days loomed in the near future, my thoughts began to race, wondering if she had any thoughts of changing her mind. If she did, I really didn't know what I would do but go into this morbid sense of depression.

But here was March, and still no phone call, thank goodness.

We signed the papers on March 7, and Amberlee Jasmine was legally ours. What a relief that there was no way she could ever go back and be taken away from us. That had always been my biggest fear with adoption. I had heard such awful stories about adoption and how they had gone so terribly wrong. But as I recall talking to Tonya during her outlandish hours of labor, she reassured me she would not do that to us. She was not going to be one of those crazy ladies who wanted their kid back on the thirtieth day. She promised me with all her heart, and she held true to that promise.

Wow, now our life could really begin.

And we started our new life, planning our family vacation with Ryan's family, going to the cabin in Colorado. We were beyond excited about taking it together.

"Do you think it is a good idea, to take her so soon?" I said, worrying about the health of Jasmine. But in all reality, she was probably the healthiest of all of us.

"Well, I think if we wait till the end of May, it won't be too cold." And so the plans began to emerge for a great time together.

The first eight weeks went by way too fast, and I had to go back to teaching. It almost broke my heart to do that, but living on one salary just wasn't going to get the bills paid, so here I was, regretting leaving Jasmine with a babysitter. Thank goodness there were only a few short weeks left in the year and then summer vacation would be here before I knew it.

It became easier to leave Jasmine with a babysitter. Not that I liked it at all, but we had no other choice. She always seemed content; it was always me everyone had to worry about. I would usually leave a tear at the door. I hated leaving her.

May was here, and the plans for the family vacation were quickly coming to a head. We had never had one together, and we were all so excited about going. Ryan's mom never really liked heights, so going through the passes would be lots of fun.

We stopped over in Raton one night to rest ourselves and give Jasmine a break in the back car seat. I can only imagine how uncomfortable she must have been.

As we made it to the cabin, we felt a peace come over us. I walked into the door, and the memories of how my family had built this cabin came rushing in. I had been only fourteen and spent an entire summer helping my dad build this house. At the time, all I wanted was to go home and be with my friends, but now that I look at the wonderful, peaceful place, I'm glad we had it to share with our family.

The cabin was nestled between many trees that enveloped it among the other homes around the area. When we built the house over twenty years ago, there were no other cabins except for maybe three others around, and now there were seven.

We unpacked the car and enjoyed five days of heavenly smells of pine, peaceful meals of fire-pit dinners, and laughter to last at least a year's worth. It was wonderful. Our family all together, and Jasmine slept through most of it, ha-ha. She, of course, was only five months old, and well, sleeping, eating, and pooping were her life, but it was so fun to watch her trying to roll over and look surprised when she did.

Life was perfect, and then we called home. And boy, did we get a surprise.

Chapter 10

W e tried to stay in communication with our family at home just to let them know how we were doing, and one night, we called our answering machine to find out whom all the messages were from and make sure there weren't any emergencies we were missing.

Well, as I listened to the machine, I heard Roger's voice, and well, he sounded concerned. "I need you to call me as soon as you get this message," said our attorney sounding deeply concerned.

I hung up the phone, and apparently, I had an ashen face because, immediately, Ryan said, "Who was that?" I didn't want to answer. As a matter of fact, I wished I had never called home.

"Roger," I said with a look in my eye that, apparently, showed panic.

"What did he want?" Ryan asked, trying to get me to talk without sounding too distressed.

"I don't know . . . He just said to call him as soon as possible. What do you think that meant?" I said, hoping something hadn't happened with our adoption. The worst things came rushing to our minds, and all we could do was just sit there and hold Jasmine, who, of course, was oblivious to everything and was smiling beautifully. *They can't have her*, I thought to myself, thinking we could run away and they would never find us, but of course, we thought better and waited for the opportunity to call Roger when we left the next day for home.

The drive home was so cruel; all we could do was think about how something was wrong with the paperwork and something got screwed up and they found some kind of loophole to jump through to get Jasmine back. I couldn't bear the thought of ever losing Jasmine. She was our life.

As we pulled into the driveway, we gave each other the look of desperation, and I knew he was thinking the same thing I was—about running away and never coming back. We took our time going into the house but eventually pushed the button on the recorder to hear the recording again. But this time, there was another message, and it was a day later, and Roger sounded even more desperate to hear from us. I couldn't help but panic as I lifted the phone and began to call him back. Maybe it was only more money. I would give everything I had, which wasn't much, to pay off whomever, but we didn't know what he wanted.

Forgetting it was Sunday, of course, the phone call went on deaf ears, and all we got was the answering machine at his office. I thought I had saved his cell phone, but I couldn't find it. We had to wait till Monday to find out the bad news. "I can't stand the wait!" I told Ryan, and I cried myself to sleep in his arms. I let Jasmine sleep in the bed next to us, thinking this might be the last time we would have her in our home. "Please, God, don't let them take her from us" was the prayer I said as I drifted off to sleep.

The next morning, we woke with Jasmine talking to us, smiling her beautiful smile, and demanding a bottle, which she vocalized quite well. I knew she was going to be a singer when she grew up because her vocal cords had no problem resounding through the entire house. Such a demanding little one, and I didn't mind catering to her especially at this moment, remembering the awaiting fate of a phone call.

It was no later than 10:00 a.m. when the ring of the phone about caused me to drop Jasmine out of the chair. "Hello," I said, wanting to cry.

"Yes, Mrs. Seevers, this is Roger. Boy, am I glad I finally got a hold of you." I didn't respond, knowing that what he was about to say to me would be the worst news I could ever hear. "Mrs. Seevers . . . are you there?" he said, thinking that perhaps I had hung up on him. And to be honest, the thought had crossed my mind.

"Yes, I am here. Is there something wrong?" I was talking with a very meek and soft voice that almost cracked when I spoke.

"Actually, I have something very serious I need to discuss with you and Ryan about Amber." *Amber,* I thought. *We call her Jasmine. Hello, hadn't he been there for the ceremony, and didn't he know we never called her Amber? Actually, Amberlee.*

"OK . . . well, she is doing great, and we just came home from vacation. That is why we couldn't call you until we got home. I'm very sorry!" I said, hoping he didn't feel ignored.

"No, I need to talk to you about Amber . . . Jasmine's biological sister!"

My whole body relaxed at that very moment, and my heart started to beat again. "So there's nothing wrong with Jasmine's adoption?"

"Absolutely not. Jasmine is yours, and there's no one or nothing ever going to talk her away from you."

I started to cry, and I held Jasmine tighter as she slept in my arms. Thank God. "OK, then what is wrong with Amber? Is she OK?" I said, remembering her sweet smile when we had first met her at Roger's office.

"Well, not really. After you adopted Jasmine, she was put into foster care, and well, she will be put into State's custody if something isn't done today," Roger said with a tentative voice. What did he mean if "something" wasn't done?

"What do you mean, *something?*" I said, almost sounding mad because I cared about what happened to the fate of Amber, not just because she was Jasmine's big sister but because she was a child, and I loved her from the moment we met her.

"Well, Deb, you and Ryan have till two this afternoon to decide if you want to adopt Amber, or she will be put into State's custody, and well . . . it's hard to get them out once they've been put into it."

And as he said the words, I almost dropped the phone. *Adopt.*

Chapter 11

In all the scenarios I had thought about happening in the conversation, this was never one I would have ever imagined. Wow, adoption, and by two. That meant we would have to find the funds etc., and we had five hours to make one of the biggest decisions of our lives. And the longer I sat there listening to the story of why she was in State's custody, the stronger my heart grew for this little person I barely knew. All I knew was, Ryan and I had enough love for a dozen kids, and well, I wouldn't want to be the one to tell Jasmine, "Well, we had the chance to adopt your sister but decided not to." To be honest, I don't think we would have ever thought of not adopting her. It never crossed my mind, but I knew I had to call Ryan before I made this rash decision by myself. "Let me call Ryan, and I will call you right back," I said as I hung up the phone and contemplated what Ryan might say.

"Hey, honey . . . got a phone call this morning," I said with a cheerful voice, but he could tell there was a hidden agenda behind my voice.

"Yeah . . . and what did he say?" he said, sounding apprehensive about what he was about to hear.

"Well, how do you feel about being a daddy again?" Silence fell over the phone, and I think he actually dropped it.

"What?"

"You heard me," I said, wishing I had told him to sit down first before I told him the news. "Jasmine's older sister, Amber, is being put up for adoption, and they have given us the first opportunity to adopt since we have her biological sister." Roger had told me Amber was in a SINK situation, which basically meant something had to be done within a certain period of time or she would be put into State's custody, and Lord only knew how long it would take to jump through all the hoops and sign all the paperwork to get her out. And as I explained the situation to Ryan, silence fell over the phone once again. I knew this had to be a lot of information to take in, and well, I was eagerly waiting.

"What do you think we should do?" he asked me, hoping we would come up with the same answer.

"I say YES," I said, with a cheer in my voice.

"Why not? What's one more mouth to feed? I don't know where we are going to come up with the money, but God can sort that out. Besides, when we met at Roger's office, I know she liked me," he said, sounding so proud of the fact that she had rather sit on his lap than on her mother's that day.

"OK. I will call Roger and get the ball rolling," I said, once again sounding beyond excited.

"Roger, this is Deb," I said, looking at my watch, knowing that it had taken Ryan and me only five minutes to decide our new future with another beautiful daughter. "We want her!"

You could tell the relief in Roger's voice as we discussed the time and date of when we would have to show up for court to sign all the paperwork and pick up Amber from the foster home there in Coffeyville. And since we had already gone through the process of adoption, the process of getting Amber would be a lot less. Wow, the mother of a five-month-old and a four-year-old, and to think less than eight months ago I contemplated if I would ever have children. God is good!

At that moment, I looked down at Jasmine, who had woken from all the excitement, and said, "Hey, beautiful, you are going to have a big sister." And I swear she smiled at me.

Chapter 12

O ur house was so not ready for a four-year-old. We needed a
bed, clothes, toys—oh my, what else did we need?

What would our parents think? I know exactly what
they would think. "Are you crazy?" But I knew deep in my heart that
this was absolutely the right thing to do. I couldn't stand the thought
of Amber spending one more night in a foster home. You hear all
sorts of horror stories about those places, and I didn't want her there
any longer than she had to be.

Roger had told us that in one week, he would have the paperwork
finished and we could go and get Amber from Coffeyville.

I began to wonder what had happened to Tonya. She had been so
animate about getting her life back on track after Jasmine had been
born, so where was she, and what was going on?

We arrived in Coffeyville at Roger's office, ready to sign any
papers we had to, to make everything legal. Amber would soon be
ours.

As we drove up to the house, it could be described as average. The lawn wasn't manicured, the shrubs around the doorway were slightly overgrown, but it looked happy. The door flew opened as we stepped onto the porch. "Where is my little sister?" Amber yelled, running into our arms. It was so wonderful to see her smiling face again. She seemed happy, and I was glad to finally have her in our arms.

"Well, she is at home with your grandparents, who you will meet too," we said, reassuring her that we still had her little sister somewhere safe. She seemed disappointed, but to be honest, that would be understandable. Apparently, the foster mother had been telling her for the past week that she was being adopted, and she would have a baby sister and a new mommy and daddy.

That was what made us the most nervous; would she accept us as her new mommy and daddy? She had been at this foster home for at least three months, and they had had a chance to groom her for her next stage in life, which meant accepting others into her life. For that, I was grateful to the foster parents, but on the other hand, all she left with was a small laundry basket with three pairs of underwear, one dress, and a few other items of clothing.

"Are you my new mommy and daddy?" she asked as, once again, she jumped in Ryan's arms, reminding us both of the first day we met her.

"Yes, we are. Is that OK with you?" we asked, hoping the answer we got would be honest and true. She nodded her head with an excited agreement.

We gathered her small box of belongings and headed for home.

"Can we eat at Burger King?" Amber asked, hoping we could take her to her favorite fast-food place. And of course, we didn't mind at all. We enjoyed a great meal together and watched her face light up when we told her she could get the kids' meal that came with a toy. She was beautiful, and she was ours.

Chapter 13

"Sissy!" Amber yelled as she walked through Ryan's folks' house. She was so ready to see her sister that she just burst through the door in search of her lost little sister. As she came around the corner of the kitchen, her face lit up like the Fourth of July, and she hugged Jasmine like she would never let her go. "Hi, I'm your big sister," she said as if Jasmine could understand a word she said, but it didn't matter. Janette and Mallory welcomed Amber with open arms just like they had Jasmine, and soon she was melting into the hearts of the entire family.

Our home was beginning to actually become a home, and it was getting closer to our first holiday together. The reason I saved this story for last was because this next and last story I am sharing was truly the day we became a family.

It was getting closer to Christmas, and Amber was beginning to act funny around us. She would begin to cry for no reason, and we were becoming more concerned about her behavior.

Christmas morning came. Ryan and I woke to the wonderful sounds of stomping feet and squealing coming from the living room, where the tree stood surrounded by presents. And as we got closer, we began to hear a faint sob coming from Amber. "What is wrong, sweetheart?" I asked, really thinking, *What could she be so upset about on Christmas morning?* For most kids, this was the day they dreamed about every year, and they couldn't wait for it to come around again. But there she was, sitting in front of the tree, crying into her little stuffed animal she was holding.

"I don't want to go!" she said faintly to herself, or maybe she was telling her animal. I'm not sure.

"Where do you plan on going?" I asked, confused by the conversation we were having on such a beautiful morning.

And as she stood up and looked at us both, she said it again, "I don't want to leave!"

"Where do you think you are going?" I asked, trying to figure out why she was so upset.

"I know I don't have too much time with you, and I don't want to go to another family. I like it here, and I don't want to go anywhere else," she said, speaking with little teardrops slowly making their way down her tiny, little cheeks. Ryan quickly responded by swinging her up in his arms, realizing she thought that we were just another stop in her journey of foster parents.

"Baby girl, you're not going anywhere. You are going to be with us forever." As she was brought back down to earth from her little trip in the air, a faint smile began to form on her face.

"You mean I don't have to leave here ever?" She was asking but not quite sure how to react.

I took her on my lap and squeezed her. "Honey, you are our little girl, and we will never let you go."

"Oh . . ." she responded, with a relieved look on her face. And at that moment, we both had realized why she had been acting the way she had for the past few weeks. She thought that she would have to go to another foster home because she never stayed at one for more than three weeks, and she had been with us for three, so far. My heart sank as I could feel the anxiety flood out of her. She was four again, and all the worries were off her tiny, little shoulders. She had been carrying that around with her, and I felt bad we never realized it before now.

"So can I open my presents now?" she asked with anticipation.

"Absolutely, but let me get Jasmine, and you can both open them up together," I told her, knowing I wanted them to share this moment together and keep it dear to their hearts.

As they ripped through paper, bubble wrap, and bows, I looked at Ryan and told him, "Miracle number 2."

Miracle 3

Often we look back on our lives and realize that every moment was a miracle of some sort. If it wasn't the time we dodged an animal in the road at the last minute, maybe it was when you found a twenty in your jeans pocket that you didn't realize you had and you were about to run out of gas and you knew there was no money in your bank account. Consider them miracles.

A miracle doesn't have to be wrapped up pretty in a bow or have this wonderful story attached to it. It's getting out of bed, making it through another day at a job you can't stand, or kissing your husband every morning, knowing he makes you smile even when he is annoying the hell out of you.

And sometimes, when you are facing problems or situations in your life, you sure wouldn't stamp *miracle* on them until maybe after you've passed through them, at least stepped back from them, and really examined what happened.

This last miracle was just that, the unexpected kind.

Miracles. Look for them. I promise you, you've had one or two in your lifetime.

Chapter 1

"**S**tand in line, and don't touch anyone, Bret!" I said, knowing that, as a preschool teacher, I could always get their attention with the "look." I loved being a teacher, and I enjoyed even more the fact that every day in pre-kindergarten was a new day. Nothing was ever the same, and well, I liked it that way. It kept me on my toes. I would never forget the time one of my little ones told me about the strange noises coming from their parents' bedroom or when I was told my head was shaped like an oval. I guess there are worse things in life, but I loved seeing their bright faces every day.

The girls were getting so big, and Amber was in eighth grade in junior high school, and Jasmine was in third grade. They were growing up so fast, and well, you know how time slips up on you and you wonder if you are doing everything you were supposed to be doing as parents. I think parenthood is trial and error, anyway. Nobody ever gets it right the first time, if ever. You just do your best and muddle through it most of the time. We would always tell the kids, "There's not a handbook for this, so you are just going to have to be patient." They never really understood what we were saying, but I figured someday they would.

Ryan, of course, was still working on the railroad, ha-ha; all the live-long day, it seemed like. I loved him dearly, and he had put up with me for fifteen years, so I know he had deserved a medal of some kind.

All was right in the world, up to this point. We had had our ups and downs, but what was about to happen would change our lives forever.

Chapter 2

"I know this may sound strange, honey, but have you had a mammogram lately?" Ryan asked me with a slight frown on his face. And actually, I hadn't had one for a very long time because, well, to be honest with you, they sucked and they hurt, so why should I torture myself with this anyway? All the posters said I didn't have to have one until I was forty, and well, I was only thirty-six, and as far as I was concerned, it could wait.

"No, not lately. Why?" I asked, trying to figure out where he was going with this.

"Well, not to put a damper on our really fun activities last night, but I noticed a lump on your right boob," he said with a little sarcasm. I had lost about thirty pounds in the recent months, so I knew that I had lost a lot of my weight in my bust section, which he, of course, was not excited about, but I figured that was part of the changes and really didn't take anything to heart.

"Well, I hadn't noticed it before," he said, sounding as if he were King Doctor and knew everything there was to know about breast exams.

"OH, stop it, you goof," I told him, thinking, *Well, he just ruined the evening for any possible midnight entertainment, hahaha.* But in the back of your mind, you always think the worse.

"The mammogram trailer will be in town next week. Why don't you just go get it checked out?" he was telling me, as if I was going to listen.

"Fine!" I told him, hoping to ease his mind off the subject. Since when did I need to worry about things like that? Good grief, I was only thirty-six, and breast cancer didn't run in my family, for crying out loud. But like a good little wifey, I decided, *What the heck?* and made the appointment.

Remember how I said the first time was a painful experience? Well, things hadn't changed much. I was actually beginning to get mad at Ryan for even making me come down here and get this stupid thing. I wanted to go and tell him, "How would you like it if I stuck your penis in the machine, smash it, tell you to hold your breath, take a picture of it, and then you could be released from the machine from hell?" There had to be a better way of doing this. But like a good wifey, once again, I did my yearly duty and left, knowing that I was done with that and didn't have to worry about it for a long time.

A few weeks passed, and so did my memory of the whole experience. What women had to go through. If it wasn't that, it was a Pap smear. God, are those awful. Open up and say AAAHHH. I think women invented colonoscopy visits to counteract the procedures women had to endure just to make the men suffer right along with us. Either way, getting older was beginning to feel like a science project, and I was the pet mouse running around the maze.

Chapter 3

The morning was a normal one. Getting the kids to get up was like raising the dead, and well, I was yelling at them to hurry up and get in the car if they wanted a ride to school. Jasmine really didn't have a choice because I had to have her at the school before seven forty-five to catch the bus to Offerle. She was definitely not my morning child.

As it felt like any other day, I received a phone call, and the office had told me that I needed to call Dr. Wray back as soon as I had a chance to. I had honestly forgotten about the tests that were taken over a week ago and really wasn't worried too much about what he had to say, so I decided to wait till lunch break. I had twenty minutes for lunch, so I quickly snuck into the office to make my phone call. "Use the phone in the back, if you want," Cathy told me as I filled her in on my last preschool story to help brighten her day.

"OK," I said, thinking this call wouldn't take long so I wouldn't be tying up the phone line very long.

"Yes, is Dr. Wray available?" I asked, knowing that perhaps he would be ready with his questions quickly.

"Debra?" I had never heard Dr. Wray sound sad on the phone.

"Yes." I was not really sure how to react to his voice.

"Well, I hate to tell you this over the phone, but according to your x-rays from last week, it shows you may have cancer . . ."

I couldn't talk, I couldn't breathe, and as the phone dropped out of my hands, I could hear him saying my name, but I couldn't answer him either.

I found myself on the floor as my world began to cave in around me. Cancer. I was going to die.

Cathy quickly ran in to the room, not realizing what I had just heard, and tried to understand why I was crying—no, not crying, sobbing uncontrollably. "What is wrong, Deb?" Cathy held me in her arms. She was always so good to me. She was actually like another mother. She always had my best interests at heart. And as I contemplated my situation, all I could say was *cancer*. Her eyes said it all.

"Where's Ryan?" she said, knowing he needed to be here with me.

"I don't know!" In the apparent rush of attention, she ran to the phone, looked up our emergency number on the computer, and called Ryan.

"Ryan, you need to get to the school immediately!" Cathy tried to tell him so as not to make him panic but was putting a little urgency in her voice, I could tell. "No, she's OK, but she needs you." I could tell he was fishing for more information. "Just get here as quickly as you can," she said, hoping he would get here soon.

"Don't worry, Deb. Ryan's on his way. He was in Offerle, so he said he could be here in about ten minutes." I was relieved that he would be here soon. "Deb, it's going to be OK . . ." But all I could do was cry. My life was ending, or it felt like it. I knew other people came into the office, but I honestly couldn't hold up my head, more or less get off the floor, but in what felt like only seconds, Ryan was holding me in his arms.

"I'll get a sub, Deb," Cathy told me as Ryan carried me out of the office. There was no way I could go back into the classroom. My heart was breaking. My children, my family—how was I going to say good-bye?

Chapter 4

Ryan took me home as I cried in his arms, wishing this entire day was a nightmare and that I would be waking from soon.

"Baby, it's going to be OK, I promise," Ryan said, hoping he could comfort me in some way. But all I could hear was *cancer* ringing in my brain. As you see others going through such awful experiences as cancer, you have a hard time putting yourself into the same positive. I sat in our lounge chair with the covers up to my chin, hoping it would all be over soon. I was so scared, and I didn't know what to do, what to say, or what to think anymore. I did know major things were about to happen, and I wasn't ready for them. You know, in the Bible, it says God will never give you more than you can handle. Well, I do believe he was on drugs when he wrote that. Just kidding. God, I felt the weight of the world was bearing down on my shoulders, and I was getting weaker and weaker as every moment passed by.

As my cell phone repeatedly kept going off, I just decided to quit answering the phone and let the answering machine take over. What was I going to tell my parents, or should I say, how was I going to tell my parents? My dad was never a man of many words, but his family always came first. And well, Mom would cry uncontrollably just like I would. I was a lot like both my parents, Mom's heart and Dad's determination. I just hoped the tenacity I had been taught as a Gilchrist would carry me through this.

I did take a call from a friend from Lewis, Kathy Lindberg, who had just recently experienced the whole cancer thing and wanted to share some of her information with me. "Deb, I know you are scared and thinking the worst, but that is exactly what the devil wants you to think. Get the facts first, make decisions with your husband, and there is always hope." She was such an inspiration to me at the moment I really needed it. Our conversation wasn't long, but long enough to bring me out of the quickly devastating ladder of depression I was descending down. We hung up after about a thirty-minute conversation, and actually, I was beginning to see a light at the end of this endless tunnel I was about to go through.

And as I was dreaming of the worst possible outcomes, I began to think about the future and what I hadn't accomplished yet. *Wait a minute!* I told myself. *I'm not dead yet, and the devil can kiss my ass. Let's go to the ball game.* And with that, I told Ryan we were going to attend our local basketball game. It was the opening season game, and I loved basketball, and I wasn't about to let a stupid thing like negative feelings keep me from it.

"Are you sure you want to do this? People are going to want to ask you questions and stuff," Ryan said, thinking that I might not have thought of that yet. But I knew that in our small town, news travels fast, and I would be on the front news of e-mails or texts being shared throughout the community. I didn't care if they were talking, but what I really needed them to do was start praying.

Chapter 5

W e walked into the gymnasium. I could begin to feel the stares, and right then and there, I knew that this was the time to face the music. Either I could cower to the feelings of fear and doubt or hold my head up high and let people know that I wasn't a quitter. "Where do you want to sit?" Ryan asked.

"Wherever?" It's funny when people know a secret about someone else and they see that person and their whispers really aren't whispers at all.

"Just ignore them," Ryan said. And I knew he wanted me as far away from the crowd as possible, and we actually sat on the visitors' side that evening. "Maybe no one will bother you over here," he said, thinking that he had me far enough away from the stares and whispers. But little did he know that people could move. I was met by many of my friends wishing me well and hoping for the best with whatever I was about to go through. You don't realize just how wonderful small towns are until you've lived in one. Our friends were just concerned, and all they wanted was to share their love for me. I could tell that Ryan was getting a little nervous from all the conversations and watching me repeat myself again and again. So we actually decided to leave the game early, but it felt good that I had overcome the urge to curl up into a ball and escape from the world, although deep down, I really wanted to do it.

The next morning, I received a phone call from Dr. Wray. "So, Dr. Wray, would you recommend Dr. Cusick?" I asked, knowing that if he had recommended her, it would be a good thing. I recall him telling me, "If you were my wife in this position, I would definitely send you to Dr. Cusick," which really made me feel good. I thought about the doctor's name and how appropriate it really was. *C* (see) *U* (you) SICK? Cusick. I thought it was pretty ironic.

But before we were to visit with the cancer doctor, I was told by Dr. Wray that I had to go to Great Bend and get a stereotactic biopsy, which in layman's terms meant "boobie-torturing machine." I thought the whole mammogram was bad; well, I was wrong. Going through that was a piece of cake compared to my next highlight of this whole experience.

As I walked into the room, I was instructed to put my boob in this hole, and the nurse was going to pull it through—through what? I do not know. I felt like a damn milking cow with my teat stuck to a machine. I had a new love and respect for milk cows at that very moment.

Anyway, after it was all said and done, I was injected with this needle I swear was twelve inches long and sounded like the loading of a shotgun when it did its thing by going into my breast one inch and pulling out whatever biopsy they needed. Thank God above for novocaine. My boob hurt so bad, and I had a hole and a bruise to prove it for the next few weeks.

I was scheduled for an appointment on December 17 to discuss the results of the test, and at that point, and she could fill in any of the missing blanks I might have had about questions and concerns we both had.

As Ryan and I were lying in bed that evening before we left for Wichita, I recalled thinking about how Ryan must feel at this moment because everything had been about me, but I knew Ryan was struggling with so much too. What was he going to do if I died? But I knew I couldn't think like that; I had to survive. He wanted so bad to do something for me, but really, there was nothing he could do but support me in any way he could. Just to hear him say he would love me no matter what meant the world. I knew my body wouldn't be the same, and I knew it might sound crazy, but I was afraid I wouldn't be the same person he had fallen in love with, or would I? I wouldn't dare bring up that subject yet, but I knew it would eventually be discussed in the near future.

The drive to Wichita was quiet, and the mood was set for an awful day. "Are you OK?" He was asking me, as if I would be in any other mood but foul.

"Yes, I'm just ready to get this over with and move on."

He was shaking his head with total agreement.

We arrived at the clinic around 10:00 a.m. and waited patiently for my appointment. I do believe Ryan read through every hunting magazine available, and I tried to figure out those impossible crossword puzzles. We were only trying to take our mind off the future. It was coming soon enough. We would know for sure if it was cancer and what we could do to stop it. This information would be ours soon.

Dr. Cusick met us at the waiting room door and ushered us into a room. "Hello, Deb. Dr. Wray has told me about your case, and we have looked at the x-rays, and I would like to have a student doctor help me examine you today." OK, great, I was going to be a test dummy for some intern.

"Whatever," I told her, acting as though I didn't care who saw me, when, in all reality, I just wanted her, but here he came anyway.

While I was lying there in my lovely paper clothing, stenograph class began. Each doctor was on both sides of me doing their doctor thing and giving each of my breasts a thorough exam. As I said before, stenograph class. And to top it off, they switched and did the same thing on the other side. It was quite a humiliating experience. I looked over at Ryan, and he had this grin on his face. And I can only imagine what he was thinking at this moment. If I knew him, it was some crazy sexual innuendo. And thank goodness it was over soon.

As they finished, Dr. Cusick put my x-ray on the screen and was looking intently at the picture. I was noticing the little white specks on one of the pictures. It actually looked like someone had sneezed on the x-ray. "What are those little specks of white, Doc?" I was asking before she realized I was watching her.

"That's it!" she said, knowing she had just given us the answer we had been dreading all day.

"Get dressed, and we will meet you in the gathering room to discuss what your options are," Dr. Cusick said urgently.

I cried in Ryan's arms for fifteen minutes, dreading what else she had for us. This was the worst day of my life.

Chapter 6

"Well, Deb, first of all, the cancer you have is ductal in situ carcinoma, and it is in the third stage." What did that mean, third stage? How many stages were there, and was that good or bad? "Basically, it's trapped within your milk duct glands, which is good." OK, I could handle the word *trapped*, which meant it wasn't anywhere else, I hoped.

"So is this a good thing?" Ryan asked with hope in his voice.

"Well, we won't know until we get in there and test her lymph nodes to see if it did get in her lymph system." I had read enough to know that once it was in the lymph system, it could be anywhere.

"So what do we need to do next?" I asked, wanting to get this out of me as soon as possible.

"We need to schedule a mastectomy as soon as possible."

Whoa, a mastectomy, I thought. "Can't you just go in and take it out without taking all of it?" I asked in desperation.

"Well, as you can see from the x-ray that there are many spots, and well, I don't want to take the chance of missing any of them," Dr. Cusick said, wanting what was best for me. "And I do believe a mastectomy would be the wisest decision to make." How could I argue with a doctor? What I also found interesting after discussing the whole situation with the doc was that she said each speck of cancer was no larger than the head of a pen, so what Ryan felt wasn't even it. God was already a part of this whole story.

I looked over at Ryan, and the first thing I thought was the fact that I wouldn't be whole anymore and that he probably wouldn't find me attractive after this. Just call me the bride of Frankenstein.

The surgery was set for January 30. Great, just a day before my thirty-seventh birthday. Happy birthday to me.

"Well, first of all, since you live so far away, I want to know if you want to elect to have plastic surgery along with my surgery." Plastic surgery—that was only for superstars and people who had extra money lying around to be used for making them look younger. Plastic surgery was the last thing on my mind, but I was trying to keep an open mind. She was hoping that if we talked to the plastic surgeon soon enough, he could get me in on the same day, and they could work together. Apparently, she sent a lot of her patients to him, and that made me feel more comfortable.

As we walked into the waiting room, a woman by the name of Andrea greeted us at the window. She was a very cheerful and lovely person. You could tell she had seen my face before from many other soon-to-be patients.

As we sat down, I began to rifle through all the literature I could get my hands on and started reading on all the procedures available. Tummy tucks, lifts, augmentation—whatever the hell that meant. I didn't know if I was ready for this information.

"Debra Seevers?" the nurse called my name, and I almost ignored her, hoping I could have an out-of-body experience at that very moment. We walked to an exam room, decorated with typical doctor stuff. I put on my favorite paper shirt and waited patiently.

Dr. Poggi seemed like a very Asian name, and what I was expecting and who actually walked in my door were two totally different people. Dr. Poggi was your typical white-collar doc, and he was actually cute, so I thought to myself, *Surely, it can't be too bad*, trying to make myself feel better about this whole thing. I'm sure Ryan was getting a kick out of the expression on my face as Dr. Poggi walked through the door. We had decided that he was going to be this chubby little Chinese dude. We were both wrong.

"Hello, my name is Joseph Poggi, and I am very good friends with Dr. Cusick. She had shared with me what she plans on performing surgically and thought you should come and visit with me. Does that sound about right?" he asked, shaking with hopeful agreement. "I know this has got to be hard, and the last thing I want to do is make it worse, but I promise you, what I do makes you feel ten times better." What did he mean by this? He began to tell us about procedures called TRAM flaps, tucks, and all sorts of things to help us decide what to do. I then got to look at some very interesting books of women's transformed boobs. I was actually quite impressed. "Holy cow!" I said after looking at this one woman's boobs, which were hanging down to her belly button. That was a little much.

"What do you want, Deb—is it OK that I call you Deb?" he said, sounding as if he had offended me. "I'll make anything you want. You deserve this," he said, making me feel like I was worth saving. All I could honestly do was sob, knowing this fate was soon to be mine. I sat in silence for as long as Ryan could stand it, and he blurted, "Pamela Anderson's. That's what she wants."

"What?" I said, punching him in the arm as fast as I could. "Shut your face, you don't have to drag the damn things around. Just make them like they were, please," I said, giving Ryan a "You say one more word and I'm going to slap you" look. He just smiled.

"Well, you weren't saying anything, and I just thought I would throw in a suggestion." Men. I swear they're either butt or boobs guys. What happened to eyes and minds? Ha-ha.

"Well, I will try to make them as close to normal as I can," said Dr. Poggi with this huge smile on his face. Normal—what was that? "I will need to take some photos before we start and decide what procedure we will be using for the surgery."

"OK," I said, thinking I wasn't ready for all this yet, but it was ready for me. And then I thought, *Pictures. How humiliating.* I felt lousy enough; I didn't need any more self-destruction going on in my life at this point.

"I promise it will be from the waist up." And he left to get his camera.

As he returned, Ryan and I had been looking through Dr. Poggi's impressive book of reconstructive masterpieces. Wow, it was amazing what plastic medicine accomplished. And now my boobs would be gracing this lovely scrapbook of memories he would be sharing with others.

"OK, Deb, I need you to take off your gown and face me." You know when you have those special dreams when you wake up going, "Really, two guys." Well, this wasn't one of them. I wasn't panting uncontrollably nor was I excited about taking my clothes off for anyone other than my husband. And to top it all off, my husband was watching this whole thing unfold before my very eyes. This was very uncomfortable, yet I realized the doc had probably seen every boob in Wichita; it still wasn't mine. Yet I got up and stood before the door, like an idiot, having him snap pictures of me.

"Deb, could you please turn around and pull your pants down on your hips?" said Dr. Poggi, wanting to get a side view of his photos. And in this brief second of divine creativity and sarcasm, I quietly leaned over and said, "Well, I'm sure glad I wore my thong today,

Doc." And in that fleeting second of power, I caused a veteran doc to excuse himself from the office, beet red. I couldn't believe I had actually embarrassed a doctor. Little did he know that I never owned a pair of thong underwear; I just wanted to give him a little crap.

He took it quite well as he walked back into the room with a smirk on his face. He looked me straight in the eye and said, "You're going to be just fine. With a positive and vivacious spirit like yours, you can beat anything, and never forget that, Deb." All I could do was smile, and he snapped a few more pictures.

In the end, we vied for a procedure that they would take my belly fat and make a boob out of it. But before we went too far with the discussion, he forewarned me that if the cancer had made it to my lymph nodes, he would not be able to perform his surgery, and I wouldn't know what happened until I would wake up the next morning.

We scheduled the next appointment before the surgery, and I was on the books in January.

Chapter 7

So far, all my holidays had been crappy this year. Thanksgiving, I found a lump; Christmas, I found out it was cancer; and well, my thirty-seventh birthday, I was going to wake up with one less part of my body. Jenny was going to be gone. Yeah, I had names for them. Actually, I didn't name them, but the fact was, Jenny was going on a permanent vacation. What I didn't realize was why they didn't seem to be in any kind of hurry. I had over a month to prepare for what was surely to be the worst nightmare yet to come, or so I thought.

But this was not just affecting me; my whole family was beginning to feel the backlash of rumors and constant negative attitudes. Amber and Jasmine were beginning to feel the pressure of what was about to happen. Many nights, we would have to sit down with the kids and hash out problems or situations that would occur at school. Sometimes other kids could be so cruel and not even realize they were doing it.

"Mom, are you going to die?" Amber asked one night when we were discussing the future.

"Absolutely not. God isn't finished with me yet," I told her, knowing I believed every word of it. Some of the kids had told her that I was going to die just because I had cancer. Try to explain that to a third grader. Jasmine was a kid who kept to herself, and often, I would find her crying herself to sleep. All I could do was hold her, letting her know that everything was going to be all right.

The month drug on for what seemed like an eternity. Teaching was very interesting, but I tried to keep it as normal as possible. I was preparing for a two-month leave of absence, and our local BB coach would be taking over. He was a tall man, and when he walked into the room, the children looked like little marshmallows, and well, that intimidation factor would work for a while until they figured out what kind of softy he really was. Derek could handle it, and if they drove him crazy, he would just take them to the gym and play. I had a feeling the kids would definitely love having him as their teacher.

As the day drew nearer, my heart grew weary, and I didn't know how to pull myself out of the slump I was in. I knew I couldn't go into the surgery with the attitude I was having, and I needed someone to give me a good wake-up call. I knew God was there, but I just needed an earthly slap in the face, and I got it from someone I never would have thought.

As I answered the phone, I heard the familiar voice, and I immediately smiled. Remember the person from the first miracle that I made sound like such an ass? Well, we had stayed friends over the years, and we checked in on each other over time.

"Hey, Gordon, it's nice to hear your voice," I said.

"I hear your surgery is coming up. Your mom was in the station the other day." Imagine that, my mom talking about me. Say it isn't so. "She said you were feeling a little in the dumps, and I just wanted to make sure you were OK." And coming from him, it sounded odd, but in all reality, many times he kept me grounded when it came to decisions from the heart. Gordon was married to a beautiful woman named Tammy with two children that were little Mini-Mes. I was so glad he had a wonderful life; that's all I had ever wanted for him. There were no longer the feelings of old, but what he did have for me was the ability to make me stop feeling sorry for myself as he said, "This isn't the Debra Gilchrist I remember! You can do this, girl. I've never met anyone more stubborn than you."

I wasn't sure how to take that, but I knew he was right. I had never given up on anything in my life, and I wasn't about to start now. "I really needed to hear that," I said with complete honesty. As the conversation lasted about ten minutes, he reassured me that everything was going to be all right. But before the conversation ended, I had to ask him one more question. "Do you think Ryan will love me as much after this is over? You do realize I will probably lose my hair and have stitches like Frankenstein?" I was crying as I said the words.

"Hey, stop it, Deb. Ryan loves you, and nothing will change that." Once again, he was bringing me back to the reality that there was hope.

"Thanks, Gordon. I really appreciate you calling." And as I hung up the phone, I knew he was right. Ryan was there for me, and I had to be strong for him.

From that day on, I think it was pure pride of accomplishing my goal—and of course, God's hand—that helped me through the next week before the big day.

I tried to start each day with a more positive attitude and began to read scriptures that would sustain my attitude throughout the day. One of my favorites came from Philippians 4:13, "I can do all things through Christ who gives me strength." And I knew I could. As long as I had family and friends who loved me and a husband who was standing by my side, nothing could rob me of my happiness. I was ready for this. Bring it on!

Some very good friends of ours kept the kids for the week while we headed for Wichita. "You listen to Aunt Deb and Uncle Troy,

OK?" They really weren't blood family, but they might as well have been. We had been through a lot together, and I knew the girls were in good hands.

We headed for Wichita the night before the surgery so we didn't have to get up at the crack of dawn, and we stayed in the motel across the street from the hospital. I was to be there at 6:00 a.m. to prep for surgery. They had also wanted me to have a special shot before the surgery began, and let me tell you, the thought of this shot made me want to pee my pants. Dr. Cusick wanted to shoot dye through my duct glands to make sure it hadn't made it to my lymph nodes, and the only way to detect this was putting it directly into my nipple. Holy hell. Are you kidding me? "Well, we will give you a shot for the pain before we give you the shot." But guess where they give you the pain shot. In the nipple. Holy hell. That experience, I have no desire to endure anytime soon.

We sat in the pre-op room, which felt like an eternity. Ryan and I hardly said a word, but then he started to talk.

"Deb, I need you to know something."

"OK," I said, wondering why all of a sudden this serious conversation.

"I know you have been worried about what you will look like when you come out of this surgery, and well . . . I just want to reassure you that I'm in love with you, not your body. I know I haven't said much this past month. I just didn't know what to say, but please know this: I love you so much, and nothing will ever change that. Do you understand what I am saying?"

Tears rolled down my cheeks. I knew what he was trying to say—that even if I came out looking like Frankenstein with a thousand stitches, well, I guess he would be cool with that. "You do realize that I will be looking like the bride of Frankenstein, don't you?" I said, trying to lighten the mood a little.

"Scars are sexy!" he said with the wide-eyed grin I had fallen in love with the first time I laid eyes on him.

"Ready, Deb?" came a voice from behind the curtain, as if on cue.

"Sure, Doc. Where's my happy juice?" I liked to call the medicine they put in my IV happy juice. It was an instant drunk, and well, I could really use one of those at this very moment.

I reached and grabbed Ryan's arm and pulled him down to me. "I will see you soon, baby. Don't worry, I'm in good hands. And always remember I love you no matter what happens." And then I was wheeled away—but wait. "STOP!" I said. "Ryan . . ." And in seconds, he was by my side again.

"What is it, baby?"

"I need a kiss for good luck." And with a roll of his beautiful eyes, he leaned down and gently kissed me.

"I'll see you soon," he said with a smile.

Chapter 8

The next thing I knew, I could hear voices, and I was aware enough to know I was still in the hospital. This wasn't a nightmare that I could wake up from. I tried to open my eyes, but for some reason, I couldn't. I knew I was awake because I could hear every conversation going on in the room. I lay there listening to my mom softly talking to the doctor, asking her questions about the surgery. And from what I could hear, it was a success.

"Why did it take so long?" I heard Ryan ask. Apparently, it had taken four more hours than they had thought.

"Well, we tested her lymph nodes, and the cancer was not found there."

A sigh of relief swept over me, not to mention the entire room. "Well, that is good, right?" Ryan said.

"Absolutely," said Dr. Cusick, "so we continued with her plastic surgery." I had remembered they had told me that if I woke up and my breast was not reconstructed, they had found cancer in my lymph system.

There was no way they could continue because the chemo I was surely going to have to take would destroy all the tissue that had been replaced in my breast area. The procedure they had done was to take the belly fat and form it where the milk duct glands would have been. So now my new name will be Belly Boob.

I reached up to feel my breast; it was there. I heard a gasping sound as my arm lifelessly fell back to my side. "Honey?" I could hear his voice, and it sounded so good to hear.

"I can't open my eyes," I said, trying to will them open, but it seemed impossible. I reached up, hoping to find the hand of someone who loved me, and I did. I could tell it was Ryan's hand, the hand that would love me through thick and thin, better or worse, stitches and scars.

"Please tell me everything is going to be OK," I said, knowing that at least there was a lump of something on my chest.

"Yes, the doctor said everything went really well." And I could tell from his voice he was telling the truth. I could faintly hear my mom sobbing somewhere in the room. I could tell it was her; I had heard that cry before. My mom was a very warmhearted woman, and she could cry at a commercial, but I couldn't say much; so did I.

"Mom, please don't cry. I'm going to be fine." And then I felt her take my other hand, and I could also feel a teardrop fall on my arm as she slowly stroked my hand.

Having my parents there was very reassuring. My dad never said much, but just having them there meant everything. He was my rock, and if I ever saw him break down, I couldn't bear to watch, so I was glad I couldn't open my eyes at that moment. I don't know if he was crying, but I know he was hurting too.

I reached down and touched my stomach first. That was what really hurt the worst. Now I know what a tummy tuck feels like, and it hurts like hell. My chest didn't really hurt too much at all, but I'm sure once the drugs wore off, that would be a whole different story.

As the morning went on, I slowly began to open my eyes, but everything was a blur. Apparently, when you have a long surgery, they put a cream on your eyes so they don't dry out. It took me a while to get all the gel out of my eyes, and then I could finally see all the family and friends who had come and supported me through all this. My dear friend Tina was there. We had been best buds since high school, and well, she had seen every stupid thing I had done in my life, and I was so glad to have her here with me again. But I knew other family members and friends would have been there, but their prayers and thoughts meant just as much as their presence.

Well, if stitches were sexy, according to my hubby, then I was the next Marilyn Monroe. I was cut, literally, from one side to the other. It looked like I'd been cut in half and then sewed back together. When I tried to stand up or lay back in my bed, boy, was the pain unbearable. I remember having a morphine drip that provided relief when needed, and I knew I pushed the little red button quite often. I swear he must have removed six inches of skin. My stomach hadn't been this flat since my skinny days of high school.

Not to mention I was looking like an octopus with four tubes for drainage hanging out everywhere, it seemed. Two were still attached to my newly formed Jenny, and the others were on each of my sides. Maneuvering around was not that easy, and getting out of bed was a feat in itself.

After lying in bed for two days, I was so nauseated by my own smell I told Ryan I had to do something, and somehow, without pulling out every stitch, I made it to the bathroom, and Ryan washed off my back. If you've ever been in bed for more than three days, you begin to develop this special scent. "eau de toilette of el stinkola," if you know what I mean. When Dr. Poggi came in one day, he even told me I stunk. Boy, that made me want to get out of there even faster.

Ryan helped me so much; there would have been no way I could have done it on my own. He was helping me do things he never would have imagined, especially after only fifteen years of marriage. Yeah, later on in life, but not yet. "For better or worse, through cleanliness and stench!" I told him as he helped me into my clean PJs.

The next few days drug on forever. Dr. Poggi told me I would be there for at least eight days, and I looked at him with my Gilchrist stubbornness and told him, "Oh no, I'm not. I'll be out of here in five." He just looked at me with the "yeah, right" look. Well, guess what? On the fifth day, I was checking out.

I had my pain prescription filled, my antinausea medicine ready, and we were headed home.

Chapter 9

People always say you can recover better at home, and I definitely knew that was true. When I stepped into our house, it was a sigh of relief; I was home. It took me almost thirty minutes to get up the stairs, but I was so grateful to get a real shower that I think I stayed in there for at least twenty minutes, just enjoying the fresh and clean feeling for as long as possible. I had to have all my tubes attached to a string around my neck, but I didn't care at that point. They were right; cleanliness is next to godliness, ha-ha.

The cards and letters began to pour in, and I couldn't tell you how much each one of them meant to me. I began to start a scrapbook with all of them in it to remind me of the love of our community. I didn't always appreciate the quick gossip train of small towns, but Kinsley's outpouring of love was one of the major factors I truly believe helped me get better. If you don't believe in sending letters of encouragement, trust me, it means the world to the person getting it.

"Hey, Mom, what do you want to eat?" Amber asked, knowing that the freezer was full of casseroles, packaged meals, and enough food for at least three weeks. I know I wouldn't lose weight sitting around the house. We had meatballs, lasagna, Tater Tot casserole, and so many more awesome meals once again provided by the many people in Kinsley and our surrounding communities. I loved little towns and the wonderful people in it.

My dad called me almost every other night, which was unusual for him, but I knew it was such a comfort for me. "How you doin', sis?" he'd always ask, knowing he would probably get the same reply but was relieved to hear it each time.

"Oh, good, tired, but one day closer to getting past this," I'd say with, hopefully, a spring in my speech. I know he never liked to see any of his kids in pain, and I never liked to show that I was ever in need, but those phone calls meant the world to me.

For the next few weeks, I had to sleep sitting up because I couldn't lie down under a 120-degree angle. When I walked, I looked like a little old lady with a bad back. And Ryan, bless his heart, every two hours would be by my side, draining the tubes that hung from my side, with Octopus Girl.

"You know, for a guy who can't stand the sight of blood, I'm doing pretty good at this," Ryan said, knowing that he got pretty squeamish at the sight of anything blood related.

"You are doing great, and I appreciate everything you have done for me," I said, thinking to myself that I wouldn't know where I would be right now if he weren't by my side.

Every day, I had to endure the mirror though. I really wished I had taken them out of my house for a while because each time I glanced in them, it was a quick reminder that things were never going to be the same. When Dr. Poggi reconstructed my breast, he didn't put a nipple on because he wanted that to heal first before any other procedures were performed. So looking at what was supposed to be a breast was quite sad. It was just a lump of flesh. A tear formed every time I looked at it, but in the back of my mind, the doc's promise kept coming back. "I'll make it as close as I can to what you have now. You'll never know you had surgery." That was a promise I was looking forward for him to keep.

Chapter 10

W ell, everything was going great, and recovery was inching along day by day. I was really missing the students, so one day, in my great insanity, I decided to go to the school and see them.

"Hey, Derek, I am going to be at the school. Could you warn the kids that I'm coming and not to let them run up to me?" I said, knowing that Derek would have them under control when I came in the door. I didn't want to take the chance hurting myself, knowing the kids wouldn't mean to, but hey, they were only kids, and well, they missed me.

"MRS. SEEVERS!" the kids yelled as I made my way slowly into the room. Immediately they stopped in their tracks. They knew something was up, and the looks on their poor little eyes was quite sad. I had lost about twenty more pounds since I had seen them last, and well, as I walked like a little hunchback, they didn't know what to do.

"It's OK, guys," I said, trying to help them make a decision on how to respond.

"Gently, one at a time, you can go give Mrs. Seevers a hug," Derek instructed them as each one, almost tiptoeing, came to me and gave me the most precious and soft hugs.

"I have missed you so much, and I know you have had a great time with Mr. Newsom, haven't you?" I said, with all of them nodding with approval. "I promise I will be back soon." And with that, the bell rang, and they prepared to go home.

It was so good to see them. It was amazing how the small hugs of children could make your entire day. I do believe that was why I loved teaching so much. And with that, Derek walked them out the door, and they headed home.

"What the hell do you think you are doing?" I heard Ryan as he was coming in the back door to my room.

"What do you mean?" I said, trying to figure out why he was so mad.

"You know those kids could have pulled out your stitches or something like that. You aren't even thinking."

And with that, I stood up and began to give Mr. Know-It-All the right act. "Listen here, I am about to go crazy in that house, and all I wanted to do was come and see the kids. I warned Derek that I was coming, and he had the kids ready to be very careful. And if you ever talk to me that way again, I will punch you in the nose. Do I make myself perfectly clear?"

Shamefully, he shook his head. "I was just worried."

"I know, but I am a big girl, and I can take care of myself." And as quickly as the argument started, it was over, and we went out to eat.

I know Derek was ready to give up the reins after a few weeks, but unfortunately, he had to be there over eight weeks, and I know the day I walked back in was the day he would take a mini vacation, ha-ha. Not only did he have to deal with four-year-olds all day, he got to go home to one every night. I know the stress level at the Newsom home had to be a little high on many occasions.

But two weeks before I walked into the classroom, I had scheduled an appointment with an oncologist in Pratt to begin my chemo treatments. We discussed the process I would have to go through before treatments would begin, and the first thing I needed was a portacath. What this little baby does is get the wonderful rat poison they put into your body just a little bit quicker by directly putting it in the artery going into the heart. This lovely procedure left this beautiful lump above my left breast.

"Doc, do I really need the Red Devil?" I said, knowing that the name said it all. "I mean, the cancer was not found in my lymph nodes, correct?"

"Well, no, it wasn't. This is just a precautionary procedure just in case any cell got away during surgery. But if you vie for the one-step-down medicine, I can't argue with you there," he said. And I was hoping, with the lesser dosage, my hair wouldn't fall out.

I had long blond hair, or at least, it was at the time. Heavens, I really didn't know what my hair color really was, but anyway, I didn't want to lose it. I know that might sound vain, but I was losing enough stuff on my body; I didn't need anything else to make me look even worse.

The lady at the hospital gave me a few wigs I could try, and I thought to myself, *I'm not going to need these.*

It was the beginning of April, and I was back into full swing of teaching. The kids weren't too excited when I told them that we wouldn't be having as much PE time as they had been having. At that point, I do believe a few asked me when Mr. Newsom was coming back. I had to chuckle under my breath.

I was taking my second treatment, and like clockwork, it took almost exactly three hours. I would sit in this specific room with at least ten comfortable lounge chairs with IV drops next to most of them. There was only one other person in there with me on most visits, but it was nice to have someone to talk to. And if I was alone, I always had Harry Potter to keep me company.

The first day after chemo was never the hardest; it was always the third. I swear I felt like every bone in my body was aching, and I could hardly get myself off the couch. I think I only took one day off from school after treatments. I was also very tired. I felt like I could sleep for days at a time. I remember I told my aide, one day, I was going to lay my head down while the kids were having center time, and I was awakened thirty minutes later with a sweet smile next to me and her asking if I was going to read them a book. "Of course, I want to read you a book." And with that, I was back up on my feet, fighting through the tiredness of cancer. But I knew I had to fight because the other thing wasn't even an option.

I remember in high school, once during a basketball game, I had twisted my ankle, and the coach had wrapped it so much that I was taped to my shoe, but I refused to come out of the game. We played six on six in Oklahoma, and well, I didn't have to move too much, but I knew giving up wasn't an option. Coach Kingery still tells me, to this day, he had never seen such determination in a player before. And to this day, I appreciate him letting me play. "Any ole nag can finish, but it takes a thoroughbred to win," he would always tell me. I was definitely not in the ole nag category, but maybe Ryan would differ on some days, ha-ha.

Chapter 11

W e were just sitting one day, watching TV, when I realized I had been playing with my hair and looked at my fingers, and strands upon strands were wrapped around my fingers. *Damn it*, I thought to myself. Maybe it wouldn't all fall out, but as the days went on, I could pick up mounds of hair off my bathroom tub each morning. I knew what had to happen.

"Hey, girls, you want to help Mom?" I yelled from the kitchen as they came barreling down the stairs. "I need a haircut, and would you like to give me one?" And with the spark in their eyes, they were in heaven. I knew it wouldn't look pretty when they were done, but I wanted them to be a part of this whole experience, not feeling like they had to be left out of anything.

"Sure, you are going to be the best Barbie doll ever!" Amber said as she brought me a doll—she had cut its hair off too—and told me that I would be even more beautiful than her hairless Barbie. Kids are so awesome. They know just what to say.

As the girls began the most interesting haircut I had ever received, I had to watch the ever-painful expressions Ryan was giving as they cut closer and closer to my ears. Pieces of hair fell off my shoulders. The thought of no hair actually made my heart jump, but to watch my girls having a great time actually made it easier. And *easier* was better at this moment in my life; I was tired of *hard*.

Ryan could take it no more, and he finally told them to stop. "I thought they were going to cut your ears off," he said with a smile of relief.

I looked at myself in the mirror and told the girls what a great job they did, and then I went into the bathroom and cried. I didn't want the kids to see my weakness, but the best still wasn't over yet. There was no way I was going to be able to go into public looking like I had mange, so Ryan finished me off with a military-style shavin'. There I stood looking in the mirror at what seemed like a stranger staring back at me.

We had called Troy and Deb over to see the new me, and being the great friend, along with Ryan, he cut his hair too. We three stood in the kitchen, looking like the Three Stooges. With a smile, I leaned over and asked Deb, "Why aren't you cutting yours?" Just joking around with her.

She just smiled and said, "I love ya, but not that much!" I told her I totally understood.

So there I was, the nippleless, hairless wonder of the world, and there Ryan stood, right beside me, telling how beautiful I was.

Adjusting to this new life was exhausting, but I knew it had to be done. Every three weeks, I was off to Pratt for my new round of rat poison and taking little catnaps in preschool. The kids started to make a game out of it, and I liked to play along. When I would close my eyes, I could hear them say, "Is she really asleep this time?" And then one would come close enough, and I would catch them as they screamed hysterically with laughter.

I even had one little boy that, over time, started growing his hair out. I would occasionally hear other boys making fun of how long his hair was, and of course, I told them to stop, but he would never tell them why. He would just say, "I am doing it for a reason." So I left it at that until one day, I saw him with a very short haircut and wondered why all of a sudden the change.

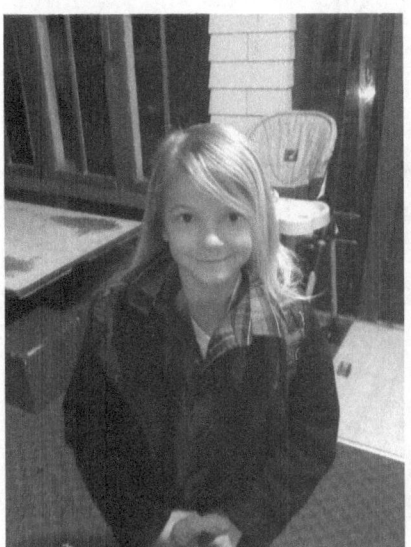 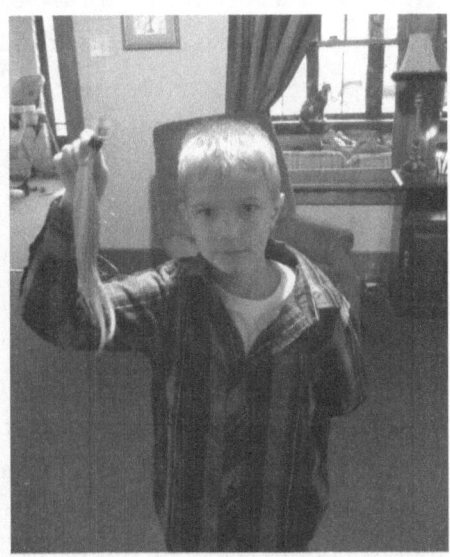

"Jaren, I like your new haircut!" I said, truthfully liking it, but I also liked his long hair too.

"I did it for you," he said with a smile.

"You did what for me, honey?" I said, trying to figure out the puzzle he was presenting to me.

"Well, after you lost your hair, I decided to grow mine out so next time you might need one, I donated my hair to make a wig for you." I could have cried right there and did later on when he wasn't around. That was one of the sweetest things anyone had ever done for me—or, at least, in behalf of me. To think, this little six-year-old waited two years to get his hair long enough so he could make a difference in the world for someone. That right there was a lesson in humility and giving. And from what I heard, he was in the process of doing it again. If something good did come from my experience, that was one I will never forget.

I also had the honor of surviving cancer with a high school student named Maria. She had been diagnosed with Hodgkin's lymphoma. And we were bald at school together. I once told her, as we walked down the hallway with our bandanas on, that everything happens for a reason; we just have to figure out what and learn from it. To this day, she is cancer-free and as beautiful as ever.

You know, sometimes we don't know why things happen, whether good or bad, in our lives. But what we do know is that you can build on them, or you can allow them to crush you from the inside out. It's not always easy to take your life back from anything like this, but I lived my life knowing that "through Christ I can do all things because He strengthens me . . . at every turn" (Philippians 4:13).

Chemo had finally finished, and I was so glad for that day. It was May and the same day the tornado hit Greensburg, Kansas. I remember this vividly because I had my treatments in Pratt and we were contemplating going to Greensburg to their local motel with an indoor pool to celebrate but decided to go on to Wichita. Like I said, miracles happen every day in our lives, and we look back thinking, *Was that my decision, or was it Christ's?*

Summer was coming soon, and I had a little peach fuzz on top, and it came back white as snow. Oh, this can't be happening. Was this actually my real hair color? I really hadn't seen it for quite some time, but surely, I wasn't salt minus the pepper already?

Harvest was only a few short weeks away, and I began telling Dad to call me when it was time. I had been driving a combine for Dad for the past several summers and looked forward to keeping the normality of my life and continue that for him. "Why don't you take this summer off?" he told me one evening. I just told him that there was NO way I was going to allow my circumstances to become a crutch to lean on, and he should have known better than to ask.

"Oh, I don't think so!" I told him. "There is nothing on earth that is going to stop me from getting on that combine this year." And with all certainty, I knew that to be true. Even if I was bald, twenty pounds less, and hated the sun because it reacted with the chemo, I was still going to be there, and I was.

My last appointment with Dr. Cusick was a relief. "No signs of cancer, Deb" were the best words I could ever hear.

Chapter 12

L ife was getting back to normal, and school was starting again, and well, I'd like to say this is the end of my journey with cancer, but it wasn't.

On my last trip to Dr. Poggi in September, just for a checkup, he discovered that a scar from my stereotactic biopsy was growing, but I didn't think anything of it. I had almost told Dr. Poggi that everything was fine and that I wasn't going to go, but Ryan insisted that I went just in case. To be honest, I'm thankful Ryan listened to the Lord's leading because if I hadn't, we wouldn't have found it again.

"Deb, I don't like the looks of that," he said, and I immediately tried to play it off like it had been there the whole time, which it had. But what I didn't realize was, cancer cells had been directly under my skin and were beginning to grow toward my lymph nodes. Right there in the office, he cut out a small biopsy and immediately had them sample it. "I don't want to frighten you, but, Deb, this doesn't look right. I just want you to be prepared." This was actually more frightening the second time because the urgency in voice really sent up red flags.

I was back at school when I got the call again. "Yes, Doctor Poggi, I understand. I will be there tomorrow morning at eight a.m." Going from finding out I had cancer and waiting thirty days to having surgery to finding it again and realizing I had less than twenty-four hours before I had to have surgery again was really scary.

I began calling all my prayer warriors, LaGayle mostly, and letting them know the situation, but there really wasn't much time to let everyone know. LaGayle is such a woman on fire for God, and if anyone had a straight shot to God's hotline, it would be her.

"Ryan, I don't think I can do this anymore," I told him, exhausted from the past twelve hours of such mental exhaustion that all I wanted to do was sleep for a week.

"You've done this once, you can do it again." He was giving me the "pull your head out of your butt" speech that I needed to hear once again. This wasn't the time to feel sorry for myself, but rather the opposite. This was not a time to sit on the bench and watch the game of life hit the fourth quarter and you forgot to use any timeouts. It was time to get into the game again.

Once again, we packed our bags, but this time, we were only there one night, and that was enough. We found out later that it was only two centimeters from my lymph nodes. You can't tell me that wasn't divine intervention.

Radiation was the option the doctors felt was the best this time, so I went to Dodge City every day for four weeks and received a pleasant little sunburn each day. I was blessed to not get the severe burns that so many fair-skinned people had received. But that experience was soon a memory too.

Actually, I began to use my experiences to help others around me and became involved with the Susan G. Komen organization in Dallas. I went with several ladies from Kinsley and Tulsa to the sixty-mile walk in Dallas for three years. Actually, I went the first time after my first bout with cancer. I walked with my fuzzy head and cramping calves. I walked all of it except for the last two miles, when my calves cramped up so bad that I couldn't stand but was so glad I did it. Thanks, Saving Second Base, Midway Style. This was the name of our team. I had *Belly Boob* put on the back of my shirts; it was definitely a conversation piece, and a lot of people learned a lot about breast cancer that year. I will never forget my experiences at Dallas. Thanks, Teri, Kathleen, and Deanna.

Do I still worry about having cancer again? Sometimes, but do I let it rule my life? Never.

Now that I've told my little world of only a few miracles, what does it all mean? Well, to you, I hope it was inspirational, and you can take courage knowing that God wants to perform a miracle in your life, and when he does, give him all the glory. And promise me that when those things that don't seem like miracles happen in your life, you will step back when they have passed and find the miracle within YOU! You are the miracle God created, so go find your story.

My prayer for you is that you look at each day as a miracle and love those around you, love life with relentless passion, and make every moment count.

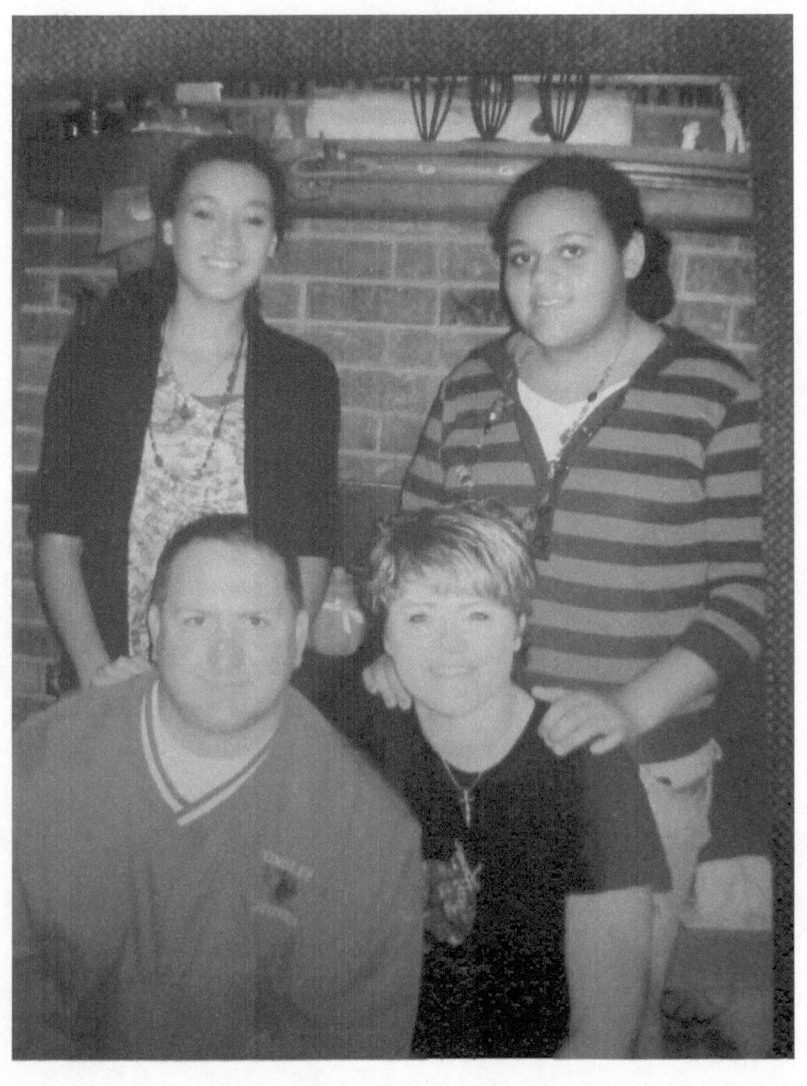

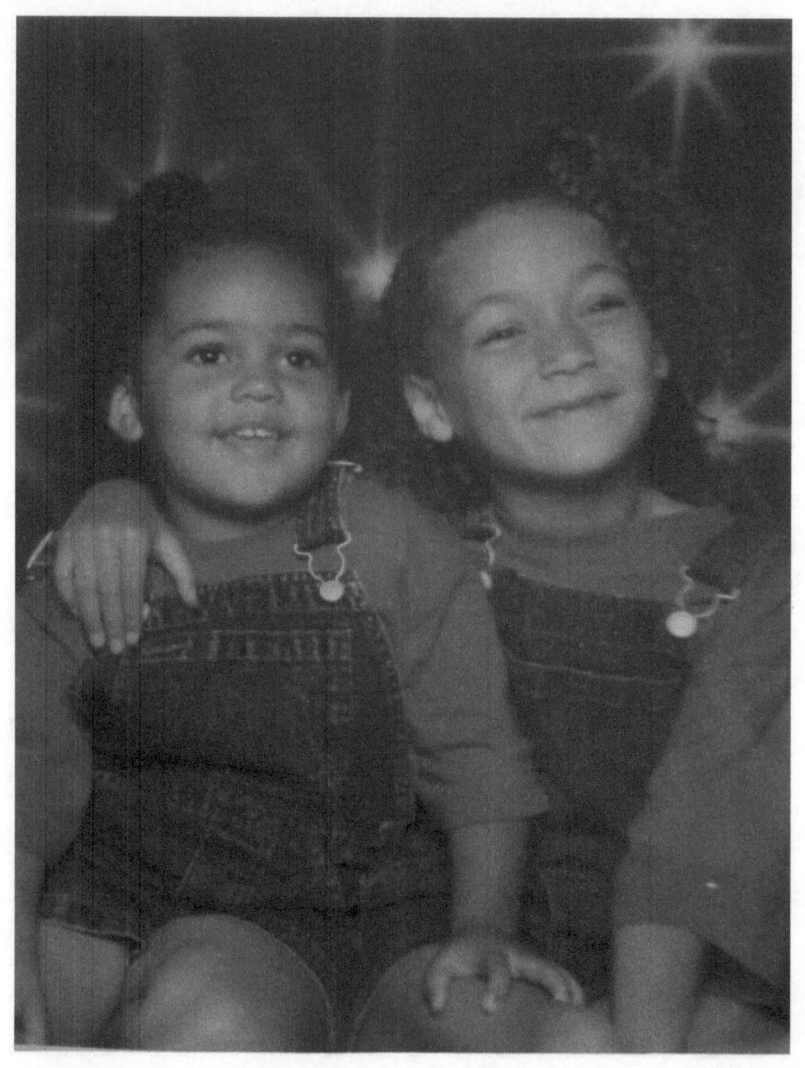

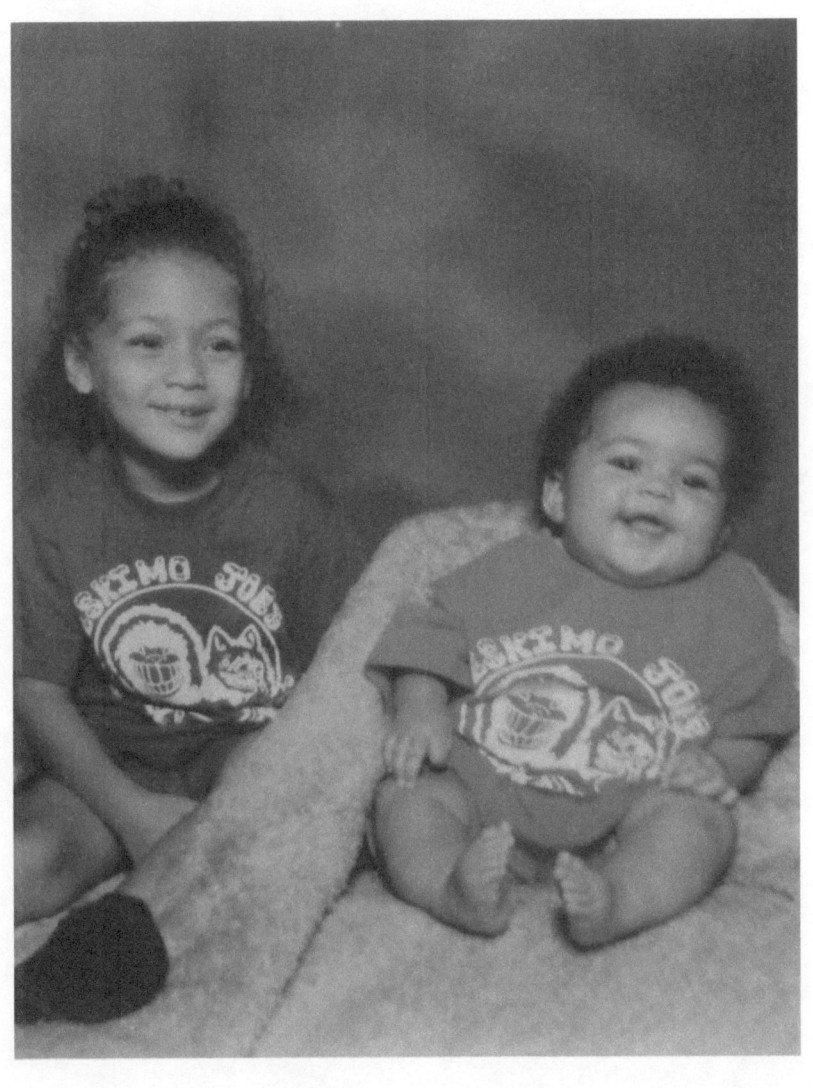